T0209429

BodyWise

Manual Therapy Is Our Ticket out of Illness, Injuries, and Pain

Mike Macy, CST, LMT

BALBOA.PRESS
A DIVISION OF HAY HOUSE

Balboa Press books may be ordered through booksellers or by contacting:

Balboa Press
A Division of Hay House
1663 Liberty Drive
Bloomington, IN 47403
www.balboapress.com
844-682-1282

Because of the dynamic nature of the Internet, any web addresses or
links contained in this book may have changed since publication and
may no longer be valid. The views expressed in this work are solely those
of the author and do not necessarily reflect the views of the publisher,
and the publisher hereby disclaims any responsibility for them.

The author of this book does not dispense medical advice or prescribe the use
of any technique as a form of treatment for physical, emotional, or medical
problems without the advice of a physician, either directly or indirectly. The
intent of the author is only to offer information of a general nature to help
you in your quest for emotional and spiritual well-being. In the event you use
any of the information in this book for yourself, which is your constitutional
right, the author and the publisher assume no responsibility for your actions.

Any people depicted in stock imagery provided by Getty Images are
models, and such images are being used for illustrative purposes only.
Certain stock imagery © Getty Images.

Print information available on the last page.

ISBN: 978-1-9822-4285-5 (sc)
ISBN: 978-1-9822-4286-2 (hc)
ISBN: 978-1-9822-4287-9 (e)

Library of Congress Control Number: 2020902463

Balboa Press rev. date: 02/08/2021

BodyWise is dedicated to the memory of
John Matthew Upledger, 1960-2017

Husband, father, son, and friend to many and former
CEO of Upledger Institute International, the Barral
Institute and the International Alliance of Healthcare
Educators (IAHE), and The Upledger Foundation.

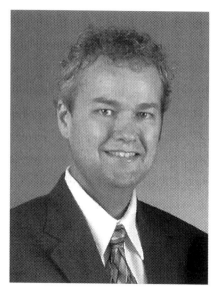

Photo courtesy of Upledger Institute International

John Matthew's healing presence and business
acumen, commitment, faith, and tireless efforts
helped spread the benefits of manual therapy to six continents.

CONTENTS

INTRODUCTION

Welcome, reader. *BodyWise* is for people who are sick, injured, or in pain and are ready to be healthy. It's also for healthy people who suspect that there's more to health than an absence of pain or illness and want to feel wonderful consistently. *BodyWise* is for those who feel that there must be more to prevention than annual physicals, tests, and imaging and that health doesn't require gobbling supplements or avoiding pleasure.

Do you have an illness that doesn't respond to pharmaceuticals? An injury that never completely healed? Was your surgery less successful than you hoped? Did it leave you less vital than before? Did a doctor tell you to learn to live with your affliction? Have you given up hope or resigned yourself to living the rest of your life at 75% or even 50% of your power? If any of the above resonates, this book is for you.

When nothing they try works, people struggling with chronic pain or illness often feel frustrated, discouraged, and even hopeless. I know because that's how I used to feel. The reason I'm so passionate about helping people with chronic illness and pain is that I've discovered that getting well can be quite simple.

I wasn't always this confident. Indeed, for much of the first 28 years of my life, I had many emotional issues as a result of childhood PTSD. But then I nearly froze to death on a solo cross-country ski trip in the Yukon. When I decided that I had at least to try to escape the trap I was in, even if it meant dying in the process, everything changed. Forty-eight hours passed from the time I made that decision until I reached an unoccupied cabin. From the very first step, I began the long transition from a passive victim to an active, healthier version of myself. In retrospect, I realized that the universe supported me every inch of the way and has ever since. I learned how to work with the body rather than against it, and that has helped me heal those issues.

Similarly, when a person has had enough pain and illness and determines to find a way out, good things start to happen. He meets a stranger who overcame a similar affliction and shares how. She runs into an old acquaintance that points her in the right direction. He stumbles upon a book and somehow opens it to a page that applies to his situation. She hears about some practitioner that specializes in treating that complaint. And so on. Call it serendipity, a prayer answered, the friendly Universe, or whatever you like. It works.

In more than three decades since my ordeal in the Yukon, I've used my experiences, thousands of hours of manual therapy training, and my understanding of language and human nature to help patients rewrite their life stories. Together, we discovered and addressed the root cause of their complaints while optimizing their body systems.

In 2017, I became the second massage therapist ever employed by the US Air Force. Considerable pressure accompanied that honor because our pain clinic was the last stop for our patients. Either we managed to reduce their pain so they could pass their physical fitness tests and resume normal duties, or their military careers were over.

To become our patients, these men and women had to pass through a gauntlet of doctors, tests, and procedures which often failed to alleviate patients' symptoms while reinforcing their worst fears. Not surprisingly, many arrived already resigned to the possibility that their problems might be permanent. Most had complex histories involving multiple injuries over years and often decades.

For me, however, these patients were ideal because I'd learned that when medicine doesn't work, the challenge is probably not biochemical but mechanical or emotional—and I'm pretty good with mechanical restrictions and the emotional content that often accompanies them.

Because my treatments were called massage therapy, patients arrived expecting a nice, relaxing massage. Imagine their disappointment when the first thing I said was that they weren't getting a massage; instead, they were going to have to roll up their sleeves and help. My next hurdle was to get them to accept manual therapy, something most had never heard of. Knowing that the work would speak for itself, I didn't waste time talking about what we were going to do other than to say that while massage might provide temporary relief, it was unlikely to find and address the root of their problems. That, I told them, was what we would do together.

Their desperation and experience following orders worked in my favor. Imagine the relief of those who after 30 or 40 minutes of therapy departed with their pain significantly reduced, occasionally halved or nearly gone. For example, one of my first patients wrote, "I nearly danced down the hallway after that first treatment." In that case, as often happens, we hadn't even touched the area of his primary complaint.

I couldn't help everyone, of course, though I tried. Most of those I couldn't help fell into one of three categories: those with major back injuries, those hoping for a medical discharge, and those who were unable to take time out to heal. I apologized to the first group and did what I could for the second and third. The lattermost were often performing the duties of several people and felt honor-bound to continue doing the same activities that had injured them in the first place even though they had bulging discs, spinal fractures, and pinched nerves. For them, light duty was not an option. They would continue to operate heavy equipment, hump big rucksacks on 20-mile forced marches and 10-mile runs, or fly around for hours on hard benches with 100 pounds of gear and parachutes strapped to their chests before the jump master sent them out the airplane's door. Before working in that clinic, I had never imagined the number of ways military personnel could get injured outside of combat. Hats off to them. The military values stoicism; unfortunately, the body does not.

I had no problem with those hoping for a medical discharge, but I soon realized that they were unlikely to report any improvement because they were attached to getting out first. The disability pay they would receive for the rest of their lives would be based on their degree of incapacity. In other words, the more disabled they were, the greater their compensation. Therefore, the last thing they wanted was to show any sign of improvement. This is nothing new. We see similar with civilians involved in personal injury and motor vehicle lawsuits and workers compensation claims.

Those ready to get better, however, and those able to abstain temporarily from punishing duties usually experienced dramatic reduction in pain and improvement in mobility. Regardless of outcomes, I am so grateful for their trust and willingness to look within. I'm thankful for having had the opportunity to help these men and women who risk their lives and health every day for me.

My faith in manual therapy stems from my own experience as a patient and 30 years as a practitioner, but those service men and women reaffirmed my belief that by finding and addressing underlying causes manual therapy can:

- Alleviate and eliminate chronic neck, shoulder, and back tension and pain
- Improve breathing, both in terms of quantity and ease
- Improve brain and Central Nervous System (CNS) function
- Improve the heart's operating conditions and function
- Resolve chronic digestive challenges
- Help patients move better and without pain
- Correct musculoskeletal imbalances that would otherwise lead to spinal fusions and joint replacements
- Improve balance, coordination, and physical performance
- Prevent injuries and falls
- Improve immune function, eliminate allergies, and resolve autoimmune challenges
- Resolve endocrine challenges
- Find and release the afflictive emotions issues, beliefs, and attitudes that lead to injuries and illness
- Regain health, and
- Improve self-esteem and position us to make healthier choices.

BodyWise explains the body's mechanical needs and how the body-mind connection affects our health. It provides the background to understand why manual therapy is so effective at resolving challenges and improving health. In many ways, *BodyWise* is an owner's manual, one we should have been given much earlier in life. It's also our ticket to lasting health because once we understand how the body works, we are positioned to make better choices about its care and maintenance.

It may be hard to believe that a pair of hands can address many of the body's most critical needs. But it's true. For example, to function properly, our internal organs require freedom from interference from neighboring tissues. The same is true with our joints, which must be free from unusual tensions to move smoothly and without pain. Blues musician John Mayall summed up the body's situation nicely: "I can't give the best I've got to give unless I've got room to move."

Furthermore, our moving must not impose tension on blood vessels and nerves, because these important structures can and will communicate that drag to the heart and brain and impair their functioning. As we shall learn, the body bends over backwards to minimize the consequences of restrictions, or tissue abnormalities, that impinge on critical organs. That compensating and those restrictions often reduce joint mobility and produce pain.

The typical adult hosts scores of restrictions from falls, collisions, infections, vaccinations, chemicals, and emotional and spiritual trauma. Remember how many times you fell or had collisions as a child, scraping your knees, elbows, hands, and shins? Even if you've never been seriously injured, many of those impacts left restrictions in your tissues. While medicine is brilliant at repairing fractures and lacerations it pretty much ignores the energy of these impacts which remain in the tissues. That's where manual therapy fits in, evicting the residual energy and resultant restrictions.

For millennia, the human hand has been part of traditional medicine everywhere. Is it currently overshadowed? Yes. However, 150 years ago, it began to emerge from the medical margins, thanks to pioneering physicians who understood the limitations of medications that often produced undesirable side effects. By embracing the scientific method, the latest research, and its own discoveries, manual therapy has become in the past 30 years a legitimate and essential branch of the healthcare tree.

The term "manual therapy" encompasses all the therapeutic techniques that rely on the human hand to treat bodily complaints. These techniques range from the most general, such as the laying on of hands, to the extremely precise, such as releasing a restriction on an artery in the brain. Well-known manual therapies include Rolfing (or Structural Integration), chiropractic and osteopathic manipulations, Alexander Technique, Feldenkrais, and various forms of massage. Manual therapy practitioners range from laypeople with minimal training to expert professionals, including physical therapists, chiropractors, medical doctors and osteopathic physicians.

This book focuses on CranioSacral Therapy and Visceral Manipulation because both 1) treat the entire body, including mind and spirit; 2) derive from osteopathic medicine and share its principles; 3) recognize the importance of mechanics and subtle motion to our overall well being; 4) are increasingly accepted by a wide variety of practitioners ranging from medical doctors to massage therapists; and 5) are increasingly available throughout the developed world.

Many of the anecdotes and claims in *BodyWise* may seem incredible to readers who have not experienced or don't understand manual therapy. Are these claims impressive? Yes. Miraculous? No, not once we understand how the body functions and how restrictions interfere with it.

If we embrace the belief that our body is defective and needs correction, we may miss our best chance at resolving challenges while at the same time running the risk of doing irreparable harm. Furthermore, a growing body of research points to the power of our thoughts in creating our experience. Therefore, if we don't like what the body is serving up, we might start by asking ourselves, "What's right about this that I'm not getting?"

When we get sick or injured, most of us expect a doctor to figure out why and make it all better. Medical options are usually limited to diagnosis, medication, or surgery. Often, however, a manual therapist can help us discover and address the underlying cause, without any unwanted side effects. The body is designed to heal. If it's not healing, the explanation may be a restriction from an old injury, infection, or buried emotion or belief.

Thanks to several brilliant physicians who were drawn to manual therapy, we now have the ideal complement for Western medicine's pharmacology, technology, surgery and psychotherapy's talking cure. The ability of highly-trained, highly-sensitive, well-intentioned human touch to find and release mechanical restrictions can help unleash our body's healing potential. Combined with Western medicine, counseling, and energy medicines like acupuncture, manual therapy positions our species to achieve levels of health only dreamed about until very recently.

BodyWise isn't an anatomy or physiology text, though it presents just enough of both so that readers can follow the discussion. In fact, some of what is most important about the body isn't taught in anatomy and physiology classes or even in medical school. Long ago, medicine opted for biochemicals and technology. In recent decades, the advances on those fronts have been astounding and saved millions of lives. Unfortunately, it largely ignores mechanics, often undercutting the body's best efforts to heal. Indeed, many health challenges may be nothing more than the body's attempt to get our attention. When that is the case, manual therapists can help us learn why and what needs to change.

Pain and illness can motivate us to look within, change our thinking, and improve how we treat ourselves and others.

Imagine the relief and joy a person can derive from making peace with the body, surmounting health challenges that had seemed permanent, and realizing that it is easy to jettison old hurts and limiting beliefs. The abatement or departure of symptoms opens doors patients might not have known existed. The light bulb of possibility flickers on, pushing away the darkness. Playing a part in birthing their relief, hope, and health has been my great privilege and reward.

BodyWise's organization is straightforward. Part One presents the principles of manual therapy. Chapter 1 introduces the philosophy behind manual therapy. Most points will sound familiar, even self-evident, though they are often forgotten. The most fundamental is the body's innate intelligence. Indeed, *BodyWise* presents dozens of examples of this intelligence and how manual therapy harnesses—rather than undermines—it.

Chapter 2 explores fascia, in many ways the most important of all connective tissue. Fascia holds us together, connects every cell in our body to every other cell, and yet magically, allows us to move. To function properly, every tissue needs the mechanical freedom fascia normally provides.

While freedom to move is critical, it is of little value if there is no movement. Chapter 3 introduces the subtle, active motions upon which our health depends. Most of us may have never heard of these motions, but it is possible to feel them and their absence.

Part Two takes up restrictions. Chapter 4 describes what they are, while Chapter 5 explains how we find them. Chapter 6 reveals how manual therapists treat them, thereby enhancing those subtle motions.

Part Three focuses on the body-mind connection, starting with its history in Chapter 7. Chapter 8 explains what the connection is and how it functions. Chapter 9 shows how we work with it, while

Chapter 10 explores the important distinction between emotional and spiritual injuries and the significance of the latter.

Part Four elaborates on the benefits of manual therapy. Chapter 11 explores nine categories of issues common to a host of health challenges. Chapter 12 explains resistance and how manual therapists work with it. Chapter 13 shows how manual therapy can prevent illness and optimize health. To further demystify manual therapy, Chapter 14 describes atypical treatment, and Chapter 15 explains how to find a manual therapist. Finally, Chapter 16 summarizes this new paradigm and the argument for working with the body rather than fighting it.

Along the way, you'll meet some of the pioneers in manual therapy and some of my patients. To respect the latter's privacy, I've concealed the patients' identities while showing you how real people have used manual therapy to regain their health. Some of their stories may seem too good to be true. They aren't.

As my patients know, health is as much a journey as a destination. I pray that all beings will experience both, but especially you. Read on!

CHAPTER 1

Intel on the Inside

Most of us ignore our bodies until a problem arises. We defer maintenance and engage in unhealthy behaviors. Then when illness or injury strike, some of us disparage the body, suggesting it is stupid. Nothing could be further from the truth. Considering everything—our food, relationships, lifestyles, toxic exposures, physical and emotional traumas, and so forth—we are lucky that the body performs as well as it does. The body's genius, evident every day, is not just theoretical. Indeed, once we understand how the body actually works, we can tap its brilliance to resolve a host of health challenges.

Intelligence in Action

Wherever we look, we see intelligence. Consider blood, for example. It flows for years without interruption, yet carries platelets that enable it to clot in seconds when we have a cut or blunt trauma so that we don't bleed out. White blood cells fight infections. Our body makes about two million red blood cells each second, which seems astounding. After 100 to 120 days, these critical oxygen carriers begin to decay, becoming increasingly toxic. The spleen removes them at the first sign of decay, but rather than waste the components, the body recycles them. How smart is that!

We needn't examine the minutiae of cellular activities to see this intelligence. The immune system is a great example. For starters, it continuously protects us from airborne and ingested pathogens by employing multiple layers of defense and defensive strategies. These include 1) physical defense, the skin and mucous membranes; 2) chemical defense, the hydrochloric acid in our stomach and immune responses like inflammation; and 3) biological defense, generalist cells like macrophages that ingest pathogens and specialized cells that kill by chemical injection. The latter can be retrained for new assignments when the initial job is done. Not yet convinced? Wondering about autoimmune challenges where the body appears to be attacking itself? Not to worry. We'll take that up in Chapter 11.

And then there is that epitome of intelligence, the nervous system. Each second, this system carries five billion neural messages. When we think of the brain, we tend to focus on the cerebral cortex—the thinking part—ignoring everything else. Talk about an oversight! A score of other Central Nervous System (CNS) structures have their own discrete functions, importance, and intelligence. For example, one of the busiest—the hypothalamus—controls metabolism, appetite, thirst, and thermoregulation automatically without needing any advice from us.

With the nervous system, we tend to focus on the nerves or neurons, as if they were the only show in town. Ironically, the neurons would die without the glial cells, which outnumber neurons nine to one. Until recently, most neuroscientists viewed the glia as mere housekeepers. There are four major types of glia in the CNS and three more in the Peripheral Nervous System (PNS). They surround neurons, hold them in place, supply them with nutrients and oxygen, insulate them from their neighbors, destroy pathogens, remove dead neurons, help make and circulate Cerebrospinal Fluid (CSF), and facilitate nerve impulse transmission. Taken together, that's some housekeeping.

However, it gets even better. In the last 30 years, researchers have discovered that glia are responsible for thinking and imagining while neurons only do reflexes, which are certainly important but far less glamorous. Discoveries like this only serve to underscore the incredible amount of intelligence packed inside us pretty much wherever we look. (For more about glia, please see Tad Wanveer's *Brain Stars: glia illuminating craniosacral therapy.*)

Intelligence in Design

Intelligence isn't limited to certain cells or cellular activities; it's also evident in the body's design. Consider the many layers and systems that protect our heart. The sternum, ribs, spine, and shoulder blades form a bony cage that protects the heart from physical trauma, while the mediastinum provides the next layer of protection. This chimney-like structure runs from the top of the thorax to the respiratory diaphragm. Housing the heart and the esophagus, the mediastinum separates the left lung from the right and protects the heart from the buffeting associated with each breath. Moving even deeper, a tough membrane called the pericardium surrounds the heart, further protecting it from mechanical impacts, pathogens, and external friction. Ligaments attaching the pericardium to the sternum and spine suspend the heart to prevent it from colliding with its bony cage. Inside the pericardial space, several layers of connective tissues separated by shock-absorbing, fluid-filled, virtual spaces defend against chemical and biological invaders and mechanical friction. Yet, despite all this protective packaging, absent injury or infection, the heart is still able to expand and contract with each heartbeat and pendulum back and forth across the chest six to eight times per minute. How smart is that!? (Chapter 3 will explain the importance of the latter.) Though the brain comes close, no other organ is so well protected. All this packaging underscores the heart's importance.

Homeostasis

If intelligence is all about the ability to solve problems, our body epitomizes the smarts. The fancy word for problem solving in living systems is homeostasis, meaning seeking or restoring a state of balance. While thought of in terms of body chemistry and pH balancing, homeostasis also includes thermoregulation, fluid regulation, energy management, repairing damaged tissues, fighting infection, and recovering from illness. Perhaps the fact that this colossal, complex endeavor proceeds continuously for most of our lives without any conscious effort or input from us partly explains our tendency to take the body for granted.

This may come as news, but we also influence homeostasis all the time. How? The body reads our conscious and unconscious thoughts. More importantly, it usually obeys them. What we think, we tend to get. For example, when we think we're coming down with a cold, we usually do. However, if we decide we're not going to get sick, we often don't. In Chapter 8, we'll learn how thoughts and feelings long buried in our tissues also influence homeostasis.

Chapter 9 explains how we can actively assist homeostasis by working directly with body structures and organs. For example, we can ask how an organ is doing, what it needs, and how we can best help it. We can even ask if it is encumbered by afflictive emotions, beliefs, and attitudes. If it is, we can give it permission to evict whatever it is.

Body Hierarchies

The fact that some tissues and functions are more important than others is another sign of the body's intelligence. Those structures and systems that protect the heart reflect its paramount importance. In the next chapter, we'll learn about the elaborate system designed to protect our tofu-like brains from blunt trauma and pathogens yet allow for the continuous changes in volume associated with CSF production and reabsorption. Next in importance come the major support organs: the lungs, liver, kidneys, spleen, blood vessels, peripheral nerves, and skin. Below them are the digestive organs, certain glands, and the musculoskeletal system. Life might not be much fun without structures like the gall bladder, spleen, or colon, but it can go on. We could argue about the details, but the notion that some structures and functions are more important than others is well accepted: doctors and other medical personnel use it constantly to save lives.

Redundancy

Redundancy implies unnecessary duplication in some contexts, but not in the body. Several critical organs come in pairs so that if one fails, we still survive. This is probably why we have two kidneys and two lungs, and why CNS structures have right and left halves, either of which can take over when its opposite is indisposed, damaged, off-line, or missing. Obviously, some critical structures don't lend themselves to duplication. For example, having two hearts would be impractical because of all the extra plumbing involved and the challenges of coordinating two heartbeats.

Given the importance of the CNS and the vulnerability of the neck, however, we shouldn't be completely surprised that the CNS's plumbing has built-in redundancies: the eft and right carotid arteries and left and right vertebral arteries. Should one side be impaired its opposite can make up the difference thanks in part two unique arterial structures inside the head. The first is the Circle of Willis, an arterial roundabout on the floor of the cranium, which receives blood from left and right carotids and distributes it to the cerebral cortex and the midbrain. Willis' circular design enables one carotid to serve both sides of the brain when the other carotid is blocked.

The second structure is the basilar artery. Formed by the confluence of the left and right vertebral arteries, this single, linear structure on the floor of the cranium supplies the three organs involved in basic life support: the pons, medulla, and cerebellum. Like the more elaborate Circle, the basilar allows one vertebral artery to supply both sides of those critical structures when the other vertebral is not functioning. This revenue sharing allowed me—and many others—to limp along for decades with only one fully functioning vertebral artery.

Design brilliance does not stop with the basilar artery and Circle of Willis. Indeed, they connect directly to each other, forming a mutual-aid system that makes the best out of any combination of challenges to the carotid and vertebral arteries. Synergistic? Yes. Brilliant? Definitely.

Exceedingly common, arterial shortfalls to the brain can result from injuries, emotional content, and internal blockages. We usually don't hear about these supply challenges because this mutual-aid system does such a good job of dealing with all but the worst cases. These vascular challenges can often be treated manually, without threading a catheter up a vein in the thigh, through the heart, and into the artery in question—and its attendant expense and risks.

Like most people, I'd never heard of the Circle of Willis and hadn't thought much about arterial restrictions until a colleague told me about losing consciousness while driving on I-80. He managed to pull onto the shoulder and stop before blacking out completely. Although the ER couldn't find anything wrong and eventually sent him home, the blackouts continued. He went from one specialist to the next trying to find their cause. All the tests and imaging came back negative: he hadn't had a stroke, Temporary Ischemic Attack (TIA) or heart attack. There was no sign of a tumor. After two years on this medical merry-go-round, he went to see Dr. John Upledger, the osteopathic physician who developed CranioSacral Therapy (CST). Dr. Upledger quickly found and released a restriction on his Circle of Willis. Problem solved: he stopped losing consciousness and was able to resume driving and return to work.

Recruitment

The fact that some organs and tissues are more important than others would be meaningless unless the body had an ability to sacrifice the less important structures and functions to protect the more important ones. Fortunately, it does: the process is called recruitment. A few minutes after a colleague improved the blood flow through my left vertebral artery, my shoulder and neck muscles relaxed. They had been recruited to minimize the arterial restriction's effects on my all-important brain. As soon as arterial service was restored, the muscle tension was no longer necessary.

Whether or not we are aware of the process or recognize the symptoms, our bodies recruit and compensate all the time. For example, after my whiplash, my neck and shoulder muscles were always rock-hard because those muscles were working overtime to protect the blood supply to my brain. I didn't know about recruitment at that time. Apparently, the chiropractors, massage therapist, and acupressure therapist who treated me didn't either. While their intentions were good, trying to get my muscles to relax and adjusting my spine was actually undercutting my body's best efforts to minimize my brain's arterial challenge. Any improvements were fleeting until a colleague finally found and addressed the underlying arterial problems years later.

Compensation

Knowing that some structures are more important than others can help us find the cause of challenges. Recruitment involves another body capacity, the ability to compensate. Think of this as built-in slack. Where none remains, structures can't compensate further and symptoms will appear, if they haven't already.

The compensatory capacity is finite and varies with the individual's history. For example, a restriction on the radial artery of the wrist could exert a drag on the heart. To protect the heart, the body will recruit muscles that draw the arm into the shoulder joint and draw the shoulder medially. Of course, if we continue to use that arm without treating the wrist restriction, we will eventually damage the shoulder joint and experience pain.

At first, if there's slack in the system, we may not even be aware of the restriction or recruitment, though we might see the resultant asymmetry between the two sides of the body in the mirror. The results of recruitment and compensation are often visible if we look for them: for example, one shoulder or hip may be higher or more forward than its opposite. Eventually, the slack will be exhausted and we may start to experience symptoms such as pain, stiffness, tingling, or visual, auditory, and chewing challenges.

Of One Mind

The following story illustrates hierarchy, recruitment, compensation, brilliance, and more. One day, I found a problem with a patient's cerebellum. Latin for "little brain," cerebellum occupies the most inferior posterior part of the brain, just above the base of the skull. Compared to his right cerebellar lobe, his left seemed shrunken, dry, lifeless. I was concerned because the cerebellum performs several critical functions.

Not surprisingly, we found restrictions in the left vertebral artery, which should be the left cerebellum's primary supplier. After releasing the restrictions, we both felt blood streaming into the left lobe of the cerebellum as if for the first time in ages. Over the next few minutes, we both felt it expand. He reported warmth, tingling, and an easing of tension in his head that he hadn't even been aware of previously. After about ten minutes, he said he could feel blood moving into his feet. This didn't surprise me. Until the brain's need for adequate arterial blood is addressed, the rest of the body will find itself short on blood. That is hierarchy at work.

Curious about what might have caused his left cerebellar issue, I asked. He said that he'd suffered a massive internal hemorrhage two years earlier. Escaping through an undetected stomach ulcer, hydrochloric acid and digestive enzymes had burnt a hole in a nearby artery. Realizing something was terribly wrong, he drove himself to the emergency room (ER) barely making it before passing out. In the ER, his heart stopped three times. With each stoppage, he was conscious of his torso and hips spontaneously arching high into the air, which struck him as bizarre. By the time the surgeons had found and patched the leak in his artery, he'd lost 26 units of blood—nearly twice the 14 pints normally on board.

Still perplexed by that arching reflex, he asked if I had any theories. I could only guess: The most obvious possibility, given his blood loss, was that the arching was his body's last-ditch effort to minimize the blood supply to less critical structures in the lower extremities and abdomen and maximize the return of what remained there to his heart, lungs, and brain. In its cleverness, his nervous system had recruited his muscles and spine to get the job done. For the two years between his three near-death experiences in the ER and his coming to see me, his basilar artery had supplied the left cerebellum with just enough blood from the right vertebral artery to keep it going.

The patient had been unaware of any symptoms of cerebellar challenges during that entire period. Yet, from what we'd both felt before and after freeing up his vertebral artery, we were both fairly confident that that left cerebellum had been more or less offline. The fact that the patient had not noticed any symptoms in two years suggests that the right cerebellum had done a good job compensating for the left's challenges and assuming its responsibilities.

I was so amazed by the story and its implications that I neglected to ask his left cerebellum how long it had been undersupplied with blood. My guess is that the left vertebral artery had been injured while the doctors were saving his life because the vertebrals are especially vulnerable to whiplash-type injuries. Another possibility: the body intentionally shut down the left vertebral to conserve what little blood remained. In any event, with its arterial well running dry, my patient's body did the one thing that would prolong its owner's life. To me, those three archings speak volumes about the brilliance built into our bodies.

Why had the doctors missed this problem after he'd been stabilized? We'll never know. The important thing is that the doctors saved his life. Had they found and addressed his arterial problem, however, we might never have heard this amazing story.

The Catbird Seat

As in real estate, so in the body. Inside the skull, there may be no better location than the Circle of Willis' neighborhood. Close by, we find the hypothalamus and pituitary, the most important components of the endocrine system and key players in homeostasis and much more. The neighborhood also includes the structures most involved in basic life support and most of the nerves of the special senses. Location, location, location.

If the blood supply to the Circle of Willis and basilar artery is sub-par, every structure in the brain will be short on blood and CSF and the critical services that both provide. We'll discuss this further in Chapter 3.

For a sense of what conditions might be like for structures closest to the Circle and the basilar artery when arterial supplies are inadequate, imagine sucking up the last drops of a drink through a straw: mostly, the result is noise, vibration, tension, and pressure. Restoring full arterial service often improves or eliminates associated challenges such as pain, ringing in the ears, and dizziness.

I Get by with a Little Help from My Friends...

The CNS's design brilliance doesn't end with the plumbing (arteries) or the bilateral nature of structures. As the previous story suggests, some structures are able to assume at least some of the duties and services normally performed by others when necessary. For example, when the temporal lobes can't perform their auditory functions, other lobes may step in to help. Thirty years ago, most neurologists viewed this neurological job-sharing with great skepticism. Today, neural plasticity as it is now known is universally accepted.

If the body is wise, it follows that it usually knows best. Therefore, our first task should be to try to understand symptoms. In our haste to help, however, we often incline toward their elimination. This approach presents several problems: we have ignored the cause, perhaps destroyed our best or only clue that a problem exists, and possibly undercut the body's efforts to minimize the problem. In the long run, we have probably exacerbated the situation.

Though simple, the principles we've touched on thus far have huge implications for treatment and prevention. For starters, while the ability to compensate allows us to survive injuries and illness, it can also obscure restrictions for years, leaving us vulnerable to relapse, re-injury, and baffling challenges. Some of that befuddlement may stem from how a restriction in one part of the body can produce symptoms elsewhere, our next topic. Readers may well wonder how we are able to feel restrictions deep in the body. That brings us to fascia.

CHAPTER 2

Fascia: Keeping It All Together

Convinced that there should be more to the practice of medicine than surgery and drugs that are often toxic, A.T. Still founded osteopathic medicine in 1874. A country doctor and Civil War surgeon, he viewed the body as a unit, with every cell connected to and in communication with every other cell. These are core osteopathic principles.

Fascia, a thin, filmy tissue, accounts for all this connectivity and communication. If you eat meat, you've met fascia, that filmy connective tissue that compartmentalizes muscles into smaller bundles. Because we don't view our food under a microscope, we might assume that fascia is limited to those stacked layers visible to the naked eye. Not true. Fascia surrounds and penetrates every cell in our body.

This continuous, nearly infinitely-layered, multi-dimensional fabric binds cells to adjacent cells and even connects intracellular organelles to each other and to the cell wall. The fascia in cell membranes allows for expansion and contraction so that muscles can change shape, size, and position as they contract and relax. In holding us together, from a subcellular level on up, fascia prevents our entire enterprise from collapsing into an amorphous blob.

Running in sheets and tubes, mostly parallel to the long axes of the body and its appendages, the fascial layers in muscles converge into thicker and thicker bundles, until they become the tendons that attach muscles to bones. Those sheets and tubes converge at joints. While providing a measure of support and stability to those joints, this arrangement also focuses forces on them, thus playing a role in joint injuries.

Fascia is often categorized on the basis of location and function. Just beneath the surface, superficial fascia anchors our skin to the deeper tissues. Deep fascia penetrates and encases the muscles, tendons, ligaments, and bones that enable skeletal movement. Visceral fascia encloses and protects our internal organs and blends with their suspensory ligaments, layers and layers of bundled fascia.

Fascia consists of two components: elastin and collagen. As its name suggests, elastin can be stretched but returns to its original size and shape after the tension is released. Given low force and sufficient time, collagen also lengthens; however, once traction is released, the collagen does not recoil. It is this putty-like distensibility that makes manual therapy possible and explains why gentle releases hold indefinitely.

In healthy fascia, the collagen fibers and sheets orient parallel to each other. Following injuries, the orientation becomes semi-circular and chaotic, and the fascia dries and thickens. This thickening adds strength but reduces elasticity and restricts movement, locally and between connecting structures. Left untreated, the thickening will restrict joint movement and eventually damage joint structures. It can also dampen the motion and vitality of our internal organs, as we'll soon learn.

While these changes are visible with an electron microscope, fascia is invisible on most imaging technologies commonly used by doctors such as X-rays, CT scans and MRIs. Therefore, even severely damaged fascia appears to be normal. Perhaps this explains why physicians frequently view those complaining of pain as head cases, hypochondriacs, malingerers, etc., a conundrum for both provider and patient.

The Medium is the Message

Far more than mere packaging, however, fascia also provides mechanical communication from one end of us to the other, independently of our nervous system. While fascia functions as a nervous system and source of mobility in primitive life forms, it functions as an auxiliary nervous system in humans, much the way a spider's web communicates the arrival of dinner, in the form of a fly, to the spider.

The following story illustrates how this works: CranioSacral and Visceral dissection classes use fresh cadavers because their tissues and bones resemble very closely those of a living person. After the dome of the skull is removed, one student gently places her hands directly on the surface of the brain and closes her eyes while another student gently tractions the cadaver's big toe until the person "listening" on the brain feels the pull. Even those queasiest about touching a cadaver brain usually overcome their qualms to experience this profound lesson in fascial connectivity.

How much fascia does the human body contain? Start with the 195,000 miles of nerves, arteries, and veins in an adult, every inch surrounded by fascia. Multiply that 195,000 miles several thousand-fold to account for all the fascial layers in and around the muscles, internal organs, and bones. In other words, there are probably billions of miles of fascia in a single body. But who's counting? The bottom line? We are all fascia all the time.

Of course, the fascial system and the nervous system are connected continuously. Indeed, fascial packaging holds nerves together, allows them to stretch and recoil, and communicates tensions to the CNS. The fascia surrounding blood vessels functions similarly, communicating tensions to the heart. Furthermore, that same fascia also communicates tension between the blood vessels and the nerves.

Fascia first entered mainstream consciousness in the United States during the presidency of John F. Kennedy Jr. Kennedy had been wounded in World War II when a Japanese destroyer collided with and sank his PT boat in the South Pacific during a moonless night. Plagued by chronic back pain thereafter, Kennedy found relief in 1955 when Janet G. Travell, MD, started injecting anesthetics into trigger points. These areas of tension within a part of a muscle produce (trigger) pain elsewhere in the same muscle, other muscles, and nearby joints. Kennedy credited Dr. Travell with making it possible for him to campaign successfully for the presidency. In gratitude for saving his political career and perhaps wanting her close at hand, Kennedy appointed Dr. Travell White House physician, making her the first woman to hold that post.

Just Add Water

Fascia also serves as a reservoir for much of the fluid in our bodies, another important and largely overlooked service from a substance generally written off as mere packaging. Called lymph, this arterial distillate cushions and protects underlying structures from mechanical force and trauma; lubricates, bathes, and nourishes tissues; and provides a hedge against dehydration. Lymph also facilitates tissues' cohesiveness and relative movement, just as a film of water holds two plates of glass together yet simultaneously allows them to slide across each other. Absent this interstitial fluid, friction increases; movement decreases; and we must work harder to move less effectively.

Though organs are sometimes classified as solid or hollow, this is only accurate in a relative sense. The body has no empty spaces. Normally, any potential space between structures is filled with fluids, gasses, ingested matter, or tissue. With the exception of our outermost layer of skin, every tissue from intracellular space on up is surrounded by lymph or serous fluid, both on the inside and outside.

Injured fascia loses some of its plasticity and elasticity. Since fascia's interconnectivity conveys this problematic situation to every other cell in the body, our well-being depends on techniques for releasing fascial restrictions and tensions and restoring normal fluid circulation and pressures. Whether the activity is walking, dancing, running, or contact sports, moving fluidly depends on normal fascial tension and hydration.

Desiccation can lock neighboring structures in a pathological dance. The tissue becomes stiff, rigid, like pasta noodles that were not stirred after they were dumped in the boiling water. Symptoms will arise eventually, both locally and on distant structures. Left untreated and unresolved, restrictions eventually become fixations, where no movement is possible.

Adhesions are cobweb-like strands of fascia formed after internal structures have been exposed to air. These exposures are common with surgeries involving open incisions, but may even occur following arthroscopic procedures because these typically involve injections of carbon dioxide gas to separate adjacent structures and provide avenues for the instruments. Of course, even the smallest arthroscopic instruments produce some fascial disturbance and desiccation. Therefore, after the incisions have healed and the risk of infection has passed, it can be helpful to manually restore normal tone, fluid pressures, and function to affected tissues.

Fascia also plays a role in immunity and communication. The associated lymph contains chemicals involved in inflammation and other immune responses, as well as neurotransmitters. Indeed, thanks to the lymph, messages travel through the fascia at the speed that sound travels through water, 750 miles per hour. This is five times faster than the speed of communication in nerves (150 mph). Injured fascia often includes injured nerves. And when nerves are injured, they often proliferate, producing hypersensitivity: Indeed, studies suggest that injured fascia can be as much as 1,000 times more sensitive to pain than normal, healthy fascia.

Fascia Giveth and Fascia Taketh Away

With fascia, communication is a two-way street. Connectivity is great when things are working well, less so when they aren't, such as when two previously independent and healthy tissues are locked together. Connectivity explains how a restriction in one part of the body can eventually drag down every other structure in the body with it. On the upside, it also allows manual therapists to follow fascial tensions to their source.

If fascia can communicate the challenges of a single cell to every other cell in the body, imagine the impact when the communication impacts the CNS. This is precisely what happened to Mary Ellen Clark, a seven-time national champion in the 10-meter platform dive and bronze medalist in the 1992 Summer Olympics. Ms. Clark had experienced vertigo occasionally throughout her career, but it resurfaced with a vengeance while she was training for the '96 Games.

Vertigo is bad enough on dry land. For a diver, it can be fatal. Mary Ellen tried herbs, acupuncture, physical therapy, chiropractic, and anti-seizure medications. She stopped drinking coffee and alcohol. Nothing worked. Doctors at the University of Miami's Balance and Dizziness Center assumed that her vertigo stemmed from the tens of thousands of impacts on her head from years of hitting the water. Their positional treatments and her sleeping in a chair for two nights after each treatment produced negligible results.

Unable to train, Ms. Clark sought the help of Dr. Upledger. Using his hands, Upledger found that fascia was transmitting tension from old knee and ankle injuries into the membranes surrounding her brain. After Upledger released those restrictions, Ms. Clark was able to resume practice just months before the Games. Despite having missed nine months of training and many competitions, she won bronze again in '96, becoming the oldest medalist in Olympic diving history. Had Upledger not been fluent in fascia, Ms. Clark would almost certainly have missed those Games.

Despite fascia's connectivity, communication, importance, and utility, the medical community largely ignores it, in part because fascia lacks glamor and is difficult to study. Anatomy books ignore fascia, too, for the simple reason that if medical illustrators showed even a fraction of the fascia normally present, it would obscure the tissues and structures they were endeavoring to show. However, as many children have discovered, the packaging is often the best gift of all. This is also true with the body. The next chapter introduces subtle motions, something else utterly dependent on normal fascial tension and hydration.

NOTE: Readers who would like to learn more about fascia might do well to visit the following website: https://www. doctorschierling.com/fascia.html.

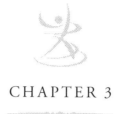

CHAPTER 3

Without Subtle Motions, There Is No Life

Out of Sight, Out of Mind

Movement is essential to health and life. Walking, talking, bending, and lifting are important, but many equally important ones are largely hidden or subtle. For example, we don't give a moment's thought to the mostly hidden movement of our arteries. However, if we look closely at the neck or wrist, we can usually see the skin move with each pulse of new blood. (A pounding or super obvious pulsing artery when a person is at rest may indicate a significant arterial restriction.) Similarly, we rarely pay any attention to another person's breathing, unless there is something seriously amiss with it. Yet in addition to supplying us with oxygen and off-loading carbon dioxide, the lungs' expansion and contraction has huge mechanical ramifications for our body, as we shall see in Chapter 11.

Most of us have a vague notion that peristalsis has to do with the propulsion of food and wastes through our digestive tract. But we don't think of our small intestine and colon "doing the wave," even though that's pretty much what peristalsis amounts to and what the colon does. Indeed, we're generally not conscious of peristalsis at all, unless and until it goes missing. Then, very soon, its absence will gain our undivided attention, as those who've experienced abdominal obstructions will attest.

Similarly, few people think about their venous and lymph returns unless there is a problem. However, many diabetics are all too familiar with the debilitating effects of the associated edema (swelling) in the feet and legs brought on by nerve degeneration and vascular disease. This pooling of stagnant fluids often leads to infection and is probably the most common cause of amputations in the US.

In any event, given the extent to which the above mentioned movements are usually off our radar, it's not surprising that most of us have never heard of visceral mobility, visceral motility, and the cranial rhythm. Yet our health and life depend on these subtle motions. When an internal organ isn't moving or a cranial bone is jammed, attention-grabbing symptoms usually alert us that something is profoundly wrong. Unfortunately, we probably will have no idea what the problem is—or how easy it can be to remedy.

My typing, your reading, and all the everyday movements that we tend to take for granted depend on the just-mentioned subtle movements at organ, tissue, cellular, and subcellular levels. These subtle movements involve matter (nutrients, neurotransmitters, wastes, solids, fluids, gasses, etc.) as well as energy, spirit, and information. Without all of these movements, there would be no life. Learning about these subtle motions will reveal why addressing the body's mechanical needs is so critical.

Mobility

Mobility includes many of the active body movements we normally think of–such as walking, running, bending, and lifting. These movements depend on muscles acting on bones, usually around joints. Joints don't exist in a void but in relationship to neighboring and transiting tissues like muscles, tendons, ligaments, and fascia. Similarly, joint function also depends heavily on the ability of nerves, blood vessels, and internal organs to relax, stretch, get out of the way, and otherwise accommodate the movement of adjacent structures. This passive mobility depends on the body having slack and is equally critical to movement and health.

Indeed, mechanical restrictions on nerves, vasculature, and internal organs often compromise musculoskeletal movements. The restriction can be at the site of musculoskeletal immobility or far from it. For example, in frozen shoulder, the shoulder is partially or completely immobilized. The syndrome can stem from a problem with the joint itself or a neighboring structure such as a lung, artery, or nerve. But it can also be due to a problem on a more distant structure like the heart, liver, gall bladder, or colon.

Take the TemporoMandibular joint (TMJ) for example. To function properly, this sliding hinge joint between the jaw and the temporal bone requires both passive and active mobility. The active movement relies on the masseter, ounce for ounce one of the body's strongest muscles. To feel the masseter, put your fingers on your cheeks and clench your teeth. The muscle should bulge under your fingers. There's a small cartilaginous disc within the joint which should passively get out of the way. If not, you may feel or hear a slight click or a louder popping. This is usually a sign of TemporoMandibular Joint Dysfunction (TMD), a potentially painful condition which can ruin a meal, conversation, or good night's sleep.

Since fascia connects every tissue to every other tissue, a particular TMD's cause could be anywhere in the body. Indeed, this is frequently the case. Fortunately, by listening to the fascia, we can track the problem to its source, as we will learn in the next chapter. For now, it's enough to know that there are two general types of mobility: active and passive.

1. Visceral Mobility

Visceral mobility is nothing more than the independent, passive ability of internal organs to accommodate the movements of neighboring structures. As previously mentioned, for example, to function properly our joints need the blood vessels and nerves transiting them to be free of restrictions so that our moving doesn't injure them. This internal freedom is critical to our health and vitality. If a nerve or blood vessel is constrained, joint movement could impart tension to the heart or brain. The body tries to minimize this tension by restricting the movement or altering how we accomplish it. Pain is the nervous system's primary way of saying, "Hey, stop it!"

Over time, in addition to feeling awkward and upsetting our aesthetic sensibilities, skewed mechanics can damage, or even destroy, the joint. We often fail to recognize what's actually going on and mistakenly assume that the lack of movement indicates a problem with the joint. As a result, we then focus our attention and therapeutic efforts on the symptoms, namely the loss of joint function and presence of pain, instead of upon finding and addressing the cause.

Generally, when an internal organ lacks mobility, we know something is amiss, though we may not know what or why. If our stomach lacks mobility, for example, our digestion will be challenged. We may experience symptoms like reflux, indigestion, and issues with our colon, but most of us won't have a clue as to the cause. Simple as it may seem, understanding visceral mobility may change your life, perhaps even save it.

A Cement Mixer

A word about nomenclature: *Many people use the noun "stomach" to refer to the entire abdomen. To avoid confusion,* *however, we use anatomical names for anatomical structures. Therefore, stomach always refers to the specific organ, which happens to be the first significant stop for food and drink making their way through our digestive tract.*

Because digestion in the stomach is as much mechanical as biochemical, the stomach perfectly illustrates the significance and complexity of visceral mobility. The mechanics begin with the three concentric layers of muscle (vertical, horizontal, and transverse) that form the stomach wall. The coordinated, vigorous contractions of these muscles accomplish the actual physical mixing of ingested food and digestive enzymes and hydrochloric acid produced in the stomach wall. The resultant homogeneous slurry is called chyme. Once the chyme is mixed sufficiently, the pylorus valve opens and those stomach muscles propel the slurry into the duodenum, the beginning of the small intestine.

Both the mixing and the expulsion/propulsion depend on the stomach's visceral mobility, which can be compromised in diverse ways. Three of the most common categories include: 1) a restriction between the stomach and a neighboring structure like the abdominal wall, respiratory diaphragm, or adjacent organ; 2) tension communicated via the esophagus, duodenum, or the greater omentum; and 3) an impingement from a neighboring structure like the liver, heart, or colon. All of these interfere with the stomach's mechanical freedom. Regardless of the cause, whenever the stomach's mobility is impeded, digestion suffers, as will the stomach's owner.

Overlook Peristalsis and the Omentum at Your Own Peril.

The stomach must also be able to passively accommodate normal body movements such as swallowing, the expansion and contraction of our heart and lungs, and less obvious movements such as peristalsis, the previously mentioned wave-like contractions in our small and large intestines that propel contents toward the anus. While the small intestine is the next organ in the digestive tract, the greater omentum provides a direct, mechanical connection between the stomach and the digestive system's last organ, the colon. Suspended from the underside of the stomach and duodenum, this curtain-like structure carries most of the blood vessels and nerves that serve the colon. Like a trampoline, the greater omentum transmits tensions to and from the stomach, small intestine, and colon. It and its neighbors can only function optimally when all those tensions are balanced. This interconnection partly explains our loss of appetite after we've had our wind knocked out physically or been sucker-punched emotionally. Either case leaves the whole system in chaos, and returning to normality can take days or weeks.

A Place for Everything

Each part of the gastrointestinal (GI) tract is designed for specific digestive processes and can only tolerate certain chemicals and enzymes. The mechanical breakdown of food begins in the mouth with chewing. Although chemical breakdown begins in the mouth with saliva, it really takes off in the stomach with the secretion of hydrochloric acid.

To better grasp the significance of visceral mobility, consider what must and must not happen once food reaches the stomach: throughout all the gastric churning just described, the valves at both ends of the stomach must remain closed to complete the mechanical mixing of food, hydrochloric acid, and digestive enzymes. Otherwise, digestion will be incomplete. The cardiac sphincter between the stomach and esophagus must remain closed to keep stomach contents and especially the hydrochloric acid from flowing backwards into the esophagus, which is not designed to handle acids and would be burned. And the pylorus valve where the stomach connects to the duodenum of the small intestine must remain closed until the stomach and hydrochloric acid have worked their magic, mechanically breaking down the food into digestible size, beginning the chemical breakdown of proteins, and neutralizing food- and fluid-borne pathogens. To remain closed when they should, both valves must be able to function independently of the stomach's contractions and anything else we might be doing like walking, bending, or lifting.

Everything in Its Place

A loss of visceral mobility is another way of saying that the stomach is stuck in position. While the degree of immobility can range from minimal to total, when the stomach lacks mobility, two outcomes are likely. First, the stomach's muscular contractions are likely to be less effective than they would be otherwise. And secondly, those contractions are likely to force one or both valves open when they should be closed. Both situations compromise digestion. The body may attempt to minimize the latter by reducing the vigor or duration of the stomach's contractions, but this still delivers an inferior product to the small intestine.

In addition, the loss of stomach mobility compromises digestion by a third avenue: mechanical interference with the digestive tract. Earlier we described how the greater omentum communicates tension across the abdomen. The omentum is attached to the lower edge of the stomach (also called the greater curve). If that corner of the fascial trampoline becomes fixed, the other components will be affected. Finally, when the stomach's visceral mobility is impaired, the stomach begins to act as a fixed axis around which neighboring structures—the esophagus, left lung, liver, spleen, pancreas, duodenum, colon, and even the spine—must move. Symptoms of impaired mobility include hiatal hernia, ulcers, respiratory challenges, spinal and rib issues, general digestive problems, heartburn, acid reflux, also known as GastroEsophageal Reflux Disease (GERD), fatigue, food sensitivities, and a tendency for food to get stuck in the esophagus. Because of our fixation on biochemistry, drugstore shelves are full of remedies for alleviating symptoms of leaky valves, when we could just as easily and more effectively treat the cause.

Most of us have experienced food getting stuck on its journey through the esophagus to the stomach. For example, in the 1990s, I was seeing a Rolfer to improve my posture, which reflected years of backpacking, kayaking, cross-country skiing, and unprocessed childhood issues. (Rolfing, aka Structural Integration, is a form of bodywork named after its creator, the late Ida Rolf.) Everything went swimmingly until after my eighth appointment when swallowed food started catching part way down.

Because I knew that the Rolfing had lengthened my trunk, and we hadn't done anything to lengthen the digestive tract, I was confident that the problem was esophageal tension. In other words, the same length of esophagus was trying to span a longer distance—thereby narrowing its opening as if the esophagus were hollow-centered rubber band. After I had shown her how, the Rolfer stretched my esophagus: problem solved, in about five minutes. No more food catching part way down.

GERD

In Western countries, between 10% and 20% of the population suffer from GERD. Reflux occurs when the cardiac sphincter (between the esophagus and stomach) fails to close completely. Not designed to handle acids, the esophagus ends up chemically burned. Unfortunately, most people haven't studied Visceral Manipulation (VM) and haven't heard about visceral mobility. Therefore, few of those who suffer from reflux realize that their challenge may be mechanical.

Also known as viscerospasms, valve malfunctions and the resultant GERD have many possible causes. Esophageal tension is one of the most common. When we are standing or sitting, gravity minimizes the backflow of stomach contents into the esophagus when the cardiac sphincter malfunctions. However, when we recline, gravity favors the backflow of gastric juices and chyme into the esophagus when the cardiac sphincter malfunctions. This is why people with GERD tend to dine early, several hours before bedtime and often sleep upright.

Reflux can be asymptomatic or excruciating. Arguably, the painful type is preferable because it drives most sufferers to treatment. Untreated, GERD can lead to esophageal cancer. Doctors usually treat GERD with medications, with varying degrees of success. Of course, the patient must continue the medication forever. Manual therapy can be highly effective for finding and resolving the underlying problems, whatever their cause, and obviate the need for medication, surgery, special diets, lifestyle changes, and sleeping upright.

While GERD is usually a mechanical problem with the valve, the cause is not always physical. The cardiac sphincter is one of five one-way valves in the GI tract that also act as emotional circuit breakers. In other words, an emotional experience can send one or more of these valves into spasm. Chapter 8 discusses this in detail. The Appendix describes how to find and self-correct these emotionally caused malfunctions.

The Ripples Go Out

In addition to affecting digestion and the GI tract, stomach mobility problems may also create physiological and mechanical challenges in other body systems. Without exhausting the possibilities, here are four common avenues by which a stomach restriction can affect the rest of the body.

1. The body may recruit (tighten) muscles in the back to minimize the problem, creating pain and spinal issues.
2. Tension may be imparted to the descending colon, approximating the left hip to the rib cage and spleen, causing respiratory, spinal, immune, neural, urogenital, and digestive challenges, eventually leading to the need for hip replacement.
3. Peripheral nerves may communicate tension directly to the spinal cord and brain, thereby affecting the nervous system.
4. Arteries, veins, and the lymphatic system may communicate tension directly to the heart, affecting the cardiovascular system.

Over time, a simple stomach restriction left untreated may produce several of these undesirable consequences and affect the entire body. Any one of the above can create spinal issues. Indeed, French researchers estimate that as much as 60% of all spinal imbalances are caused by restrictions on more important structures such as arteries and internal organs.

Repetitive Motion—Compounded Continuously

In the last 30 years, the concept of repetitive motion injuries has become widely recognized. Of these, the best known is carpal tunnel syndrome—a painful and debilitating irritation of the median nerve named after the tunnel-like joint in the wrist through which the nerve passes. In severe cases, excruciating pain plagues the entire arm continuously. In those situations, sleep will also be problematic, leaving the patient exhausted and often depressed and defeated.

A leading cause of surgery in the US, carpal tunnel is common among those involved in repetitive activities like word processing, data entry, mail sorting, component assembly, food processing, farming, and commercial fishing. The human body is not designed for repeating the exact same skeletal motion thousands of times a day, day in and day out, for weeks, months, even years. Production quotas, time constraints, financial pressures, hostile supervisors and co-workers, pre-existing injuries and conditions, and improper body mechanics exacerbate the problem. The irritation accumulates.

As numerous as these occupational motions may be, most are trifling compared to some of the ongoing movements in the body that we tend to overlook, like our breathing and heartbeat. Indeed, both of those unavoidable motions probably exacerbate carpal tunnel symptoms.

And the Beat Goes on

If we aren't accustomed to viewing the body mechanically, we may find it hard to appreciate the significance of a slight loss of visceral mobility in an internal organ. While we can imagine how a restriction on the stomach or esophagus could impede digestion and create GERD and other issues, quantifying the significance of a given restriction presents more of a challenge. To gain a better sense, let's consider our perpetual motion organs, the heart and lungs.

It may not seem like the volumetric change associated with the heartbeat would have a large effect on neighboring organs. Absent mechanical restrictions, that might be correct. But all of us have mechanical restrictions. Here, a little math helps. At 72 times per minute, on average, the heart beats nearly 104,000 times per day and 38 million times per year—more when we exert ourselves or have hypertension. As you might imagine, being stuck in a position where something was continuously nudging or tugging even slightly on you might prove irritating. Indeed, even a fraction of those 38 million nudges from the heart might throw a stomach with even a small restriction off its feed. Way off.

Unfortunately, it doesn't end there. In the same scenario, the heart has to work a little harder on each heartbeat to compensate for the elevated resistance coming from the stomach. Over time, extra work may translate into hypertension and possibly shorten the life of the heart or some critical connecting structure, like the aorta. In other words, a restriction on the stomach or some other internal organ might eventually lead to an aortal rupture, which is almost always fatal.

Breathe Not a Word

Likewise, at an average 12 respirations per minute, the lungs inflate about 17,000 times per day, and 6.3 million times a year. Compared to that of a heartbeat, the number of repetitions may be only a fraction, but the movements associated with normal breathing are comparatively large, and not just for the thorax. Inhalation can impact the neck, lower back, abdominal organs, and the brain. In patients with significant lung restrictions, I might feel both legs pull up into the hip sockets on each inhalation. Could lung restrictions destroy hip joints and lead to replacement surgery? Over a period of decades, absolutely.

It's also worth remembering that shortness of breath may originate in the lung or thorax but could just as easily come from restrictions on some neighboring structure such as the heart, liver, diaphragm, stomach, or elsewhere. For example, the psoas muscle runs from the transverse processes of the lumbar vertebrae to the uppermost, innermost part of our femur. The psoas assists with the contraction of our respiratory diaphragm. During normal inhalations, the psoas contracts an inch and a half. When we breathe deeply, during exertion for example, the psoas shortens four inches! This is but one avenue by which a lung restriction could affect the kidneys and lower back.

Or vice-versa: the kidneys ride on the psoases. Among the body's most important organs and on par with the lungs in the body's hierarchy, the kidneys eliminate toxins and maintain the fluid and electrolyte balances so critical to blood chemistry and heart function. Therefore, the body will go to great lengths to avoid irritating the kidneys. Should a kidney lack mobility because it is stuck to the psoas, we will not be able to breathe as deeply as we should. Speaking of shallow breathing, Chapter 11 explains how stress results in our unconsciously tightening our respiratory diaphragm, and Appendix A provides a simple and effective exercise to reverse the process.

To compensate for lung restrictions, we'll breathe more shallowly and shift the effort to the pleural domes, the uppermost portion of each lung. Also called neck breathing, the latter can interfere with the arteries that supply the brain and arms and the brachial plexus, a nerve switchyard in the lower neck that serves the arms, thorax, and abdomen. Shallow breathing and neck breathing result in suboptimal gas exchange and will eventually damage our spine.

Here's some food for thought: many of my patients present with lung restrictions. (I know because I can feel the effects of these restrictions on each inhalation.) Two factors account for the prevalence of lung restrictions, the sheer volume of air we breathe and the variety and ubiquity of causes. However, most of those patients are unaware of their lung restrictions, unless they smoke or have a history of respiratory challenges. Many factors account for this lack of awareness, including our tendency to quickly become accustomed to the new situation. At 720 breaths an hour, a slight decrease in aerobic capacity usually escapes our awareness or is quickly forgotten. However, with each restriction we release, the typical response is, "Wow! I can breathe better!" Or "Wow! I had no idea I couldn't breathe!"

Mountains from Molehills

Most patients are also oblivious to the consequences of lung restrictions, even endurance athletes. This is not meant as a criticism, just a fact. For example, an athlete came to me complaining of severe pain in the upper left abdomen. Months earlier, his transverse and descending colon had torn loose from its hanger under the spleen, collapsed on itself and created a life-threatening bowel obstruction. Emergency surgery to re-suspend the colon had eliminated the obstruction but not the associated pain.

This patient was one heck of a belly-breather: on each inhalation, his belly distended hugely as if he'd swallowed a cantaloupe. He hoped I'd be able to reduce the pain near his surgery site long enough for him to complete a 110-mile ski marathon. My intuition told me his pain had to be related to his belly-breathing, but I failed to find the connection.

He survived his race and returned a year later with the same complaint, just before his next ski marathon. I saw the connection as soon as he removed his coat. Remember, he was an Olympic-caliber belly-breather. The fabric of his shirt spiraled 75 degrees clockwise on each inhalation, mirroring what was going on deep in his chest. His entire left chest expanded, but not his right. Because of a restriction behind his right breast, his right lung barely inflated. The spiraling focused force just below the left ribs, precisely where his transverse and descending colon had torn loose from its hanger under the spleen. As soon as we released the restriction, mobilized his right lung, and rebalanced both, his pain eased.

Adding Insult to Injury

The foregoing story typifies the domino-like effects stemming from restrictions in general, and especially the lungs where movements are so large. To obtain sufficient air on each inhalation when lung restrictions are present, the body enlists secondary breathing muscles in the shoulders, neck, and lower back. As a result, each inhalation compresses the lumbar vertebrae on the sacrum and pile-drives the head on the neck, compressing the cervical vertebrae. Lung restrictions produce chronic muscle tension, pain, headaches, and migraines. Eventually one can expect bone spurs, disc and vertebral damage, and compression of the brain stem. The brain stem will compress the midbrain and eventually all CNS structures which will affect every system in the body.

Given the prevalence of lung restrictions, no wonder spinal surgeries are so common. Many spinal challenges reflect the cumulative toll of 6.3 million large, repetitive motions a year, year after year in the presence of significant restrictions. (Because lung restrictions are such a major source of health challenges, we'll return to them in Chapter 11.) Furthermore, no wonder spinal surgery only addresses spinal pain about 50% of the time.

The situation is even more complicated and the implications even more significant because, as we are about to learn, our organ function and vitality also depend on another type of subtle movement, visceral motility.

Visceral Motility

In addition to needing to move passively, all internal organs need to move actively around their own internal axes. This active motion is called visceral motility. Motility is an inherent, continuous, back and forth motion, unique to each organ and independent of other structures.

Dr. Jean-Pierre Barral, a French osteopath, first described visceral motility. In the 1970s, while working as a respiratory therapist in a lung hospital in the Alps, Barral noticed that lung diseases also affected the abdominal organs. When a patient dramatically improved between treatments, Barral asked him what he'd done. The patient explained that he'd been treated by a folk healer. Barral found the healer and began to study his techniques. This eventually led to his discovery of visceral motility.

Typically, visceral motility is a cyclical rotation of an organ around an internal axis unique to that organ. With abdominal viscera and the lungs, motility consists of two phases. In *inspir*, the organ moves superior-lateral-posterior (upward, outward, backward). In *expir*, the organ returns inferior-medial-anterior (downward, inward, forward).

Most organ motilities are paired. Paired organs include right and left lungs, right and left kidneys, ascending and descending colon, and liver and stomach. Motilities of pairs should be synchronized and balanced in quality and amplitude so as not to interfere with each other or adjacent structures. The heart's motility is unique in that it isn't paired with any other organ;

instead, it swings back and forth across the thorax like a pendulum in an old-fashioned clock. Any restriction that impedes the heart's motility decreases the heart's efficiency, makes it work harder, accelerates wear and tear, and most likely shortens its life.

Just as the accuracy of a mechanical clock depends on the synchronized and uninterrupted movement of all the gears in the clock's interior, our health depends on all these unseen motilities deep inside us. To function properly, all internal organs—including the bladder, uterus, glands, blood vessels, nerves, and brain—need both mobility and motility.

Wake of the Unseen Object

Most of us have seen the wake of a fish swimming unseen beneath the surface. But few of us can claim to have actually seen the motility of any organ. That presents a question: how do we know that visceral motility is real? For starters, we can feel motility—through the body wall— with our hands. And how do we know we aren't just imagining the movement and then tricking our hands into feeling it?

Using modern imaging techniques, Dr. Barral and his colleagues have documented motility. Furthermore, this same technology shows significant, lasting improvements in motility following manual therapy. Most importantly, the improved mobility and motility have eliminated symptoms and illness and enhanced organ function and vitality.

Why haven't you heard about visceral motility before? For starters, motility is subtle. Furthermore, medicine is so focused on biochemistry and pathology that most physicians don't give much thought to motions, subtle or otherwise. But that will change. Indeed, European osteopathic colleges now require all students to train in VM for six months.

In any event, just as we showed how stomach function depends on mobility and the unimpeded contraction and relaxation of its muscles and valves, the stomach's vitality and efficiency also depend on motility. Restoring its motility gives the stomach one heck of an energetic jumpstart. More importantly, since the techniques used to obtain it are gentle, improved motility tends to last indefinitely, barring new trauma or overlooked restrictions.

Cumulative Impacts

Motilities are palpable for two reasons. First, the human hand is highly sensitive—and grows significantly more so with training and practice. And second, the movements involved are measurable, and not just in nanometers and millimeters, but in centimeters and inches. Motilities are continuous and independent of heartbeat and breathing. Varying from person to person, they run between six to eight cycles per minute.

Since motilities are supposed to continue without interruption, a fully motile organ travels enormous distances. For example, in an adult, the liver weighs about seven pounds, making it our heaviest internal organ. The motility of a restriction-free liver amounts to as much as three centimeters—about 1.2 inches—in each direction per cycle. With over 17,000 cycles per day, the mileage accumulates quickly: indeed, a fully-motile liver travels almost 600 meters, or a lap and a half around a standard running track, per day! The body must have good reasons to heave our liver 100 miles or more each year. It does: motility is critical to the function and vitality of each organ, and therefore to our overall health and vitality.

Moving from the Gross to the Sublime

In addition to organ motilities, some manual therapists can even detect sub-motilities within the functional units of "solid" internal organs like the liver and kidneys, enabling them to zero in on and treat problems with nearly surgical precision and minimal risk to the patient.

If you've seen videos of cellular activities under a microscope, you probably aren't all that surprised to learn that there are subtle movements like organ motilities going on in our bodies. From microscopy, for example, we know that individual cells move continuously relative to adjacent cells and structures and that these movements are of vital importance to cellular metabolism and well-being. In fact, the microscope shows so much movement within and between cells that living tissue looks like it has the heebie-jeebies and appears to be more fluid than solid.

Indeed, even the most solid parts of us, our bones, aren't as solid as we think. For example, we know that the cells in our leg bones move slightly, relative to each other, with each step we take. The polarity of each bone cell changes with each step, as well. We are designed this way: otherwise our bones might rapidly disintegrate under the constant pounding associated with walking and running. In gravity, the exact opposite occurs: constant loading and unloading actually strengthens bones, while a lack of loading leads to bone loss and osteoporosis.

If our experience with bones is limited to the long-dead bones of skeletons in biology class or at the butcher's, this may seem startling, even impossible. But living bones are altogether different from dead. Living bone is flexible, malleable, plastic. Indeed, bones continuously reshape themselves in response to how we load them, or don't. If you want strong bones, load them daily. Exercise!

Now that we have a basic understanding of visceral mobility and motility, let's consider another critical, if subtle, tissue movement, one that originates in our CNS but that reverberates through every tissue and cell in the body.

Cranial Rhythm

The Cranial Rhythm (CR) is arguably the most important of all the body's subtle motions on account of its relationship to the CNS and by extension everything else. The CR is wholly separate from heartbeat, breathing, visceral mobility and motility, and brain waves and varies from individual to individual. For most people, the rate will be somewhere between eight to 12 cycles per minute.

The CR stems from the pulse-like creation and constant reabsorption of Cerebrospinal Fluid (CSF) inside our head. All fluids resist compression. Similarly, our soft, tofu-like brains and their associated blood vessels don't like to be compressed either. Therefore, something has to give to accommodate the continuously changing volume of CSF. What gives are the bones of the cranium which separate during the CSF creation phase and approximate during reabsorption. Spent CSF is reabsorbed continually by structures in the intracranial membranes. With production rates approximately double those of reabsorption, the continuous reabsorption balances the intermittent production over the course of each cycle

Ideally, barring restrictions, these movements follow prescribed paths. For example, the frontal, occipital, and temporal bones rotate around a horizontal axis running from ear to ear. At the top of our head, the parietals rotate around another horizontal, fore and aft axis, sliding laterally and inferiorly away from the crown, like the retractable roof of an astronomical observatory dome.

A Mind of Its Own

While the rhythm is most pronounced in the head, the entire body widens and shortens during the CSF creation phase and narrows and lengthens during CSF reabsorption, thus honoring the law of the conservation of mass. Cranial rhythms are most readily perceived at the occiput (the bone at the back of the head) and at the sacrum (the large bone at the base of the spine) but can be felt anywhere. That's correct; don't be fooled by the name: the cranial rhythm is palpable throughout the entire body.

Practitioners describe the vitality of a person's cranial rhythm according to its symmetry, quality, amplitude, and rate. Symmetry refers to equality between the distance traveled during the expansion and contraction phases. Quality refers to whether the motion is smooth, sticky, or jerky. Amplitude relates to whether the motion seems minimal or large. Rate involves the number of cycles per minute.

One convenient place to feel the cranial rhythm is on the feet of someone lying on their back: each leg and foot should roll laterally-medially-laterally around an axis running through each leg from hip to heel. Discrepancies in the rhythm from one side of the body to the other and from one area of the body to another are common and indicate the presence of restrictions. To feel your own cranial rhythm, sit comfortably in a chair or on a stool, place your hands very lightly on your thighs, relax, don't think, breathe, and allow the motion to come into your hands.

Although a few medications and illegal substances dampen rates and quality, weak cranial rhythms usually result from restrictions. These restrictions could originate from anywhere in the body, not just from within the confines of the CranioSacral System (CSS). Releasing the restriction can restore a full, powerful cranial rhythm to an area or tissue where, a moment before, the rhythm was almost imperceptible.

The fact that the cranial rhythm manifests throughout the body makes it doubly useful, for both assessment and treatment. Asymmetries in the rhythm from place to place make it possible to detect and pinpoint restrictions. The hydraulic forces associated with the cranial rhythm also facilitate releases, making many nearly effortless. Indeed, thanks to those forces, on occasion simply finding a restriction may be all that is needed for its release. Failing that, the CSS's hydraulics, the therapist's intention, and various tricks of the trade usually prevail.

In any event, CranioSacral Therapy (CST) is always done without force. The therapist begins with zero pressure and adds a gram at a time up to a total of five (5) grams, the weight of a nickel, until the tissue responds. If the underlying tissue resists, the therapist meets the resistance exactly and, if necessary, gradually adds pressure, up to an additional five grams. Combining this gentle pressure with a ton of intention, the therapist waits for the tissues to change.

Though in some places such as on the feet they may feel many times larger, cranial motions amount at most to a millimeter or two, which explains why most of us never notice our own or another person's cranial motions. Nonetheless, we can learn to perceive these movements and their absence. Although we may not be consciously aware of cranial motions, some of us may notice more than we realize; however, lacking context or encouragement, we may tend to ignore our senses, file away the perception, and never get back to it. I've had several experiences that suggest that before learning to ignore subtle motions like the cranial rhythm, infants, children, cats, dogs, and even horses probably notice them, as the following anecdote suggests.

"Is He Dead?"

Years ago, I was giving free CranioSacral mini-treatments at a health fair in a mall. A patient lay on his back, face-up, on my massage table, in a "still point." This means that his cranial rhythm had stopped. This is not uncommon. Indeed, without any outside assistance, the cranial rhythm stops briefly for maintenance and repair off and on throughout the day. This occurs spontaneously in the absence of a practitioner. However, on this occasion, I'd intentionally induced a still point to help the patient's body integrate the work we'd just done.

A young boy approached and whispered something in my ear so softly that I couldn't understand what he was saying. I had to ask him to repeat himself three times. On the fourth try, I finally heard, "Is he dead?"

I was floored, and impressed. No wonder the boy had lowered his voice: he'd noticed the quality of the patient's stillness, and it had scared him. This eight-year-old had perceived something significant that none of the other passersby had, namely that the patient's cranial rhythm had stopped. The man on the table was profoundly—though thankfully not terminally—still.

The boy maintained his vigil until after the man sat up, thanked me, and walked away. The fear and confusions on the boy's face gradually dissipated as I congratulated him for being so observant and explained why this man had seemed dead. Not entirely convinced, the boy slowly moved off, trying to fathom what that profound stillness meant. In my dreams, he's become a gifted physician, with an open, questioning mind and a skilled manual therapist.

Still Points

The importance of the cranial rhythm cannot be overstated. For starters, the function and vitality of our CNS depends on the cranial rhythm and the associated circulation of CSF, as we shall soon see. When any significant healing or repair happens anywhere in the body, the cranial rhythm shuts down temporarily. These timeouts for reorganization and recalibration have no unwanted side effects and are entirely therapeutic. Inducing still points is only problematic when there is swelling inside the cranium. A recent brain bleed, stroke, concussion, or CNS infection are the only contraindications.

In the Beginning...

In 1911, a young osteopathic physician discovered the cranial rhythm. Examining human skulls, William Sutherland, DO, noticed that the sutures (joints) between the various cranial bones varied in design. For example, the sutures between the frontal and parietal bones interlocked as did the joint between the left and right parietals. In contrast, the joints between the temporal and parietal bones overlapped and were beveled.

Starting from the osteopathic principle that form follows function, Sutherland theorized that these designs reflected the motions possible at each joint. For example, interlocking can only accommodate separation and return, while a beveled joint can accommodate sliding in two planes. Today, we know he was correct.

Investigating further, Sutherland was able to feel these motions on his patients and assumed that they were significant. As a scientist and physician, however, he needed certainty. Therefore, he fitted a leather football helmet with adjustable thumbscrews. Wearing the helmet and using himself as the test subject, he tightened certain screws to stop the motion of a single cranial bone. Then, leaving the screws in place for hours, he would go about his day and note the results.

Sutherland found that, when immobilized, each bone produced discrete physical and behavioral symptoms. Many of these were unpleasant, some debilitating, and a few produced disturbing behaviors. However, Sutherland soon had an extensive catalog of symptoms associated with each cranial bone restriction. Subsequently, when a patient would appear with a particular symptom, Sutherland had a good idea of which bones to check and treat. After nearly twenty years of research, clinical treatments, technique refinement, and collaboration with a select few colleagues, he finally published his results.

Born under a Bad Sign

By then, Sutherland and his associates had become known as the Cranial Osteopaths. In Sutherland's day, American and British medical schools taught that the cranial bones fused in late adolescence. Craving acceptance as equals by medical doctors, few osteopaths were willing to challenge this fundamental medical precept. Instead, the larger osteopathic community did what they could to ignore and silence Sutherland and his colleagues.

By its very nature, dogma tends to resist discussion. This was the case with the notion that cranial bones fuse in late adolescence. Despite the lack of concrete evidence or scientific studies or data, denial came easily because, to casual observers, the joints of cadaver skulls appear to be fused, just the way the earth can appear to be flat, even when we know it isn't. Furthermore, the skulls in question were dried. The bones had long since lost their plasticity and ability to move.

Sutherland believed that CSF was manufactured solely in specialized structures in the cranium called choroid plexi. This theory prevailed until recent years when huge advances in imaging techniques revealed that CSF also filters from capillaries directly into ependymal glial cells in the brain. In other words, the blood-brain barrier is not a single structure, as the term suggests, but a special property of the brain's capillaries, glial cells, and choroid plexi which allow only certain types of molecules to pass, presumably based on size.

Is Now and Ever Shall Be

In the US, change came slowly. While assisting during a neurosurgery in 1973, Dr. John Upledger, a young osteopath encountered an unfamiliar rhythm. According to American medical theory at that time, his job was quite simple: immobilize the spinal cord while the surgeon excised plaque deposits from its surface. It was also a little anxiety provoking because a slip of the scalpel could nick the dura and leave the patient paralyzed or dead. Therefore, Upledger took his role very seriously. Imagine his horror and the neurosurgeon's consternation when the dural tube—the spinal cord's tough covering—would not cooperate. Despite Upledger's best efforts, the tube moved continuously Having never heard of such a thing and being a scientist, Upledger had the presence of mind to check the monitors, which showed that this mysterious, rhythmical pulse was independent of the patient's heartbeat and breathing.

Somehow the neurosurgeon managed to complete the excision without nicking the spinal cord. Everyone recovered, including the patient, Upledger's professional ego, and his relationship with the neurosurgeon. Intrigued, Upledger knew what he'd seen was real. Suspecting it was important, he was determined to find out.

After much reflection, he vaguely recalled attending a lecture on cranial osteopathy toward the end of his osteopathic schooling.

This memory sent Upledger searching the literature for articles on cranial osteopathy. He concluded that what had so complicated his surgical assignment was the cranial rhythm that William Sutherland had described. Wondering why most physicians don't notice this rhythm, Upledger assumed it was because it was so subtle. Furthermore, he realized that most neurosurgeons wouldn't notice it because their first incision into the cranial dura instantly depressurized the system, thereby eliminating the pulse, which would remain off or imperceptible until after the hole was patched at the end of the procedure.

Science Will Out

The more Upledger learned, the more he was convinced that he'd stumbled onto something significant, and the more he wanted to know. Unfortunately, the larger osteopathic community was still suppressing cranial osteopathy in hopes of gaining full acceptance with medical doctors. Nonetheless, Upledger managed to secure federal funding from the National Institutes of Health for a multi-year, multi-disciplinary study at Michigan State University School of Osteopathic Medicine to determine once and for all if the cranial rhythm actually existed and, if so, how it worked.

Upledger was able to document the rhythmic widening and narrowing of the sutures. Using electron microscopes and tissue samples from the cranial bones of fresh—as opposed to preserved—cadavers, Dr. Upledger and his colleagues discovered nerves crossing the joint between the left and right parietal bones at the top of the head. Since these nerves were stretch receptors, he theorized that they helped regulate CSF production.

According to this theory, during the CSF production phase, the parietals separate until these nerves signal that it's time to stop CSF production. Absent production, CSF reabsorption continues, and the parietals begin to come back together. Upledger theorized that when the joint narrowed sufficiently other nerves called for the resumption of CSF production. He called this the pressure-stat model because it had the effect of maintaining stable fluid pressure inside the cranium.

Upledger and his research team subsequently documented and measured cranial rhythms in patients of all ages. They confirmed many of William Sutherland's discoveries and unraveled some of the associated mysteries.

Nothing New under the Sun

Upledger published his results and became an ardent proponent of the CranioSacral System (CSS). Sensing the system's vast therapeutic potential, he talked to anyone who would listen. Eventually, that led to a presentation to an association of medical doctors in Israel. Expecting hostile questions but hearing no response at the end of his presentation, he began all over again. His host politely interrupted, suggesting that the audience needed no convincing. This was old hat to them, the Israeli explained; Italian medical doctors had known about all this since before World War II and had carried their knowledge to Israel immediately after. Upledger had been preaching to the choir.

Shifting Gears

Thereafter, Upledger spent less energy trying to convince the medical establishment and more effort developing and disseminating CranioSacral Therapy (CST), making numerous remarkable discoveries along the way.

While doing his research at Michigan State (MSU), Upledger had been eager to explore CranioSacral Therapy's clinical applications. What he needed were some willing patients. There happened to be a home for autistic children just down the road from MSU. At the time, there was even more fear and ignorance about mental conditions than there is today. As a result, autistic children were routinely institutionalized and abandoned by families and society. When Upledger approached the managers to see if they would allow him to work on the children, they were overjoyed. Almost no one wanted anything to do with these kids.

Most children suffering from autism tend to shrink from human touch and communication, especially from strangers. Initially, these kids were no different, hiding under tables and desks to avoid Dr. Upledger. Since he could induce a still point from anywhere on the body, Upledger was able to surmount this challenge by touching a single foot, ankle, or hand—whatever he could reach. Autistic kids tend to be extremely sensitive, and they liked what they were feeling: namely extremely neutral, non-judgmental, safe touch. Within a very few visits, the children were racing each other to the door to greet him and be the first to be treated. Upledger and the kids' caretakers soon saw astounding changes in the aspects and behaviors of these children.

Based on those results and his experiences in the clinic, Upledger made some quick calculations. The conclusion was inescapable: even if every osteopath devoted all his working hours to giving CranioSacral treatments, he would never be able to satisfy demand. Therefore, Upledger began to teach CST to nurses, massage therapists, other medical practitioners, and anyone else interested.

Either not realizing how gentle Upledger's cranial techniques were, or concerned that the public might confuse these lay people with osteopathic physicians, numerous osteopaths opposed his efforts. To be sure, some osteopathic manipulations are indeed forceful and, in untrained hands, potentially harmful. But Upledger wasn't teaching osteopathic manipulations. He was teaching essentially zero-force techniques, most of which had no contraindications.

CST's effectiveness carried the day. Taking his lumps from the profession, Upledger persisted and prevailed: today, more than 125,000 healthcare practitioners worldwide have at least some training in CST and allied modalities like Visceral Manipulation. Thousands more laypeople provide basic services for friends and family members.

The CranioSacral System

What's in a name? The word CranioSacral stems from the fact that the sacrum moves in sync with cranial bones, and specifically the occiput. Thanks to Drs. Sutherland and Upledger and their colleagues, the CSS is now widely recognized as an important physiological system. It meets the medical definition of a system: namely, it consists of multiple tissues and structures all working together to perform a service, in this case, one of the most essential services in the entire body: protecting, nourishing, oxygenating, managing waste, and basic housekeeping for the CNS.

System components include:

- The cranial bones and sacrum
- The intracranial membranes
- The membranes surrounding and protecting the skull and spinal cord

- The structures involved with CSF production, circulation, and reabsorption, and
- CSF and its distinctive rhythm.

The CSS's components provide suites of services. For example, a single, elaborate, three-part structure, the intracranial membranes:

- Hold the cranial bones together
- Divided the brain into right, left, upper, and lower hemispheres
- Contain sinuses or cavities that collect and remove spent CSF and blood, and
- Connect and communicate with the membranes lining the cranium and the spinal cord.

This structure-within-a-structure is further evidence of the intelligence in mammalian design. For example, the CSF cushions the brain and spinal cord from shock by floating the brain and spinal cord in a virtual sea. The buoying alone is life-sustaining. The average brain weighs about 1350 grams—almost three pounds. *In situ*, buoyed by adequate CSF, that same three-pound brain weighs a mere 57 grams, approximately an eighth of a pound and one twenty-fifth of its actual weight. Absent this flotation, our mushy brains would be quickly crushed by their own weight.

CSF also delivers oxygen, immune cells and nutrients and whisks away debris and toxins. CSF can even chelate (remove) heavy metals from the brain for processing by the kidneys, liver, and elimination by the colon, bladder, lungs, and skin. Any shortage of CSF or impediment to its circulation will impair brain function.

It may be helpful to think of the CSS as the CNS's innkeeper, providing every service we associate with a modern hotel:

reception, bellhop, concierge, security, HVAC, communications, messaging, room service, housekeeping, plumbing, electrical, and waste management. In other words, without the CSS there would be nothing, no CNS, no life.

First among Equals

While we could argue at length about whether the heart or the brain is more important, the existence of the CSS certainly reflects the importance of the CNS. While the heart's packaging, which we described in Chapter 1, is extremely complex and impressive, it is not normally considered a separate physiological system, but a major component of the circulatory system, which is a subset of the cardiovascular system. The first chapter explored the brilliance built into the body's design and function. The existence of the CSS and its relationship with the CNS should erase any lingering doubts on that score.

More than a century ago, the temporal bones' constant in-and-out motion reminded Dr. Sutherland of the fanning gills of a fish. As a result, Sutherland referred to the CSS as the Primary Respiratory System (PRS). Given the CNS's importance and the CSS's role in oxygenating the brain, the primary respiratory label remains appropriate today. Happily, the phrase has not gone completely out of use. SacroOccipital Technique (SOT) chiropractic also calls the CSS the PRS.

New Appreciation for an Old Friend

In 2013, researchers at the University of Rochester announced that in lab mice whose sleep patterns were experimentally disrupted, CSF production and circulation was significantly reduced. This reduction resulted in accelerated accumulation of some of the same toxins in the mice craniums associated with Alzheimer's and dementia in humans. Other studies show that, in the absence of therapeutic intervention, CSF production and circulation decreases about 50% in people between the ages of 40 and 60 years old. Given the increase in longevity, stress, and environmental pollution, no wonder the incidence of Alzheimer's, dementia, Parkinson's, and other CNS diseases is increasing.

Doubting Thomases

Today, more than forty-five years after Dr. Upledger and his associates proved the existence of the cranial rhythm and the CSS, pockets of resistance to CranioSacral Therapy persist in the larger medical community even though nobody has ever challenged the original research methodology or findings. The resistance seems mostly driven by adherence to the old belief that the bones of the skull fuse in adulthood, and there are always those who insist that anything cannot be proven in double blind clinical trials is voodoo. (These trials may be the standard for testing drugs but, for obvious reasons, don't lend themselves to the testing of manual therapies.) Similarly, some resistance is semantic, based on the belief that if it doesn't involve drugs or surgery, it isn't medicine. Generally, manual therapists understand the distinction between the practice of medicine, which focuses on the diagnosis and treatment of disease, and using the human hand to find and release restrictions so that the body can function better.

In science, new theories are often initially met with skepticism, then rabid hostility, and finally with ho-hum, what-else-is-new, tell-us-something-we-don't-know matter-of-factness. I'd like to think that we're nearing the end of that process. Misguided folks can cast aspersions, but their efforts to protect the public from what they view as "quackery" result in millions of people suffering needlessly. Tens of millions of patients have benefitted from CST and VM and other manual therapies, overcoming many conditions for which traditional medicine offers only diagnosis, management, or no hope at all. We're about to explore in greater detail how all of this works.

It's not every day that a scientist discovers a brand-new physiological system. For example, the endocrine system was discovered in the 1690s and the immune system in 1796. Discovering something as important as the CSS and identifying its components, processes, and function is a big deal. Outside of Osteopathic circles, William Sutherland never received the credit his discoveries deserve. His immense contribution to the prevention and treatment of disease is only now beginning to be recognized. Although Dr. Upledger had a very successful career and has helped train tens of thousands of manual therapists, his and Dr. Barral's contributions to healthcare deserve much greater recognition.

Conclusion

There are other subtle motions in the body besides the ones discussed above. For example, there are tidal motions associated with the circulation of lymph, energetic movements associated with acupuncture meridians and chakras, and subtle movements in our bones. The ones we've explored, however, are the most important mechanical motions.

Having discussed visceral mobility and motility, and the cranial rhythm and the CSS, we can now turn our attention to treatments and learn how practitioners find and release restrictions, restore mobility, motility, and cranial rhythms and how these treatments eliminate pain and unleash our healing potential.

CHAPTER 4

Restrictions

Restrictions are areas of increased friction, density, entropy and decreased elasticity, fluid exchange, motion, and vitality. Categorized musculoskeletal, craniosacral, or visceral based on the tissue in which they occur, restrictions can be within a single tissue, such as in an arterial wall, or between neighboring structures, such as between the liver and the respiratory diaphragm.

Initially, most restrictions produce relatively minor changes with localized effects. Absent treatment, however, the changes become more significant and their effects spread, owing to fascial connectivity. Given enough time, what began as a small restriction can affect the entire body. Being denser than healthy tissue of the same type, restrictions also tend to collect additional traumas. In this sense, they can become the health equivalent of black holes.

The trend with restrictions is toward absolute immobility, at which point we call it a fixation, where all traffic stops—fluid, blood, nutrients, and energy. Furthermore, fixations become axes around which everything else must move. Long before a restriction becomes a fixation, however, it will have been disturbing surrounding structures.

Fortunately, we needn't be students of the human form to recognize fixations when we see them. Watching someone with a fixation doing something as familiar as walking or jogging can disturb our sense of how bodies should move. Even if they aren't in pain, we may find their awkwardness upsetting. Indeed, we may describe such movements as "mechanical". This is ironic, given, that their restrictions render normal movements and mechanics impossible.

Restrictions are pathological; in other words, they cause disease. The decreased fluid exchange results in the build-up of metabolic wastes and toxins. This build-up in turn may cause tissue death and even lead to cancer. A particular restriction's significance depends on its degree, location, duration, and the body's compensatory reserve. Generally, the more complete the restriction, the more important the structure involved, and the longer the duration, the more serious its impact. Fortunately, almost all restrictions can be treated; therefore, the vast majority of these consequences are preventable.

Multiple Causes, Similar Results

Restrictions result from infections, vaccinations, surgeries, dentistry, and physical, chemical, thermal, emotional, and spiritual trauma. Decades may pass between the onset of a restriction and the appearance of a symptom. In the interim, however, the disruption of normal body mechanics and function consumes increasing amounts of energy.

In Utero and Birth Trauma

Pregnancy and birth often produce restrictions because the developing tissues are exceedingly delicate and thus easily injured. These restrictions are particularly insidious because the young nervous system needs to develop so rapidly that a given disturbance or delay has significantly greater consequences—both short- and long-term—than it would for an adolescent or adult. Furthermore, even during normal labor and delivery, mechanisms of injury abound: the mother's pelvic bones; the baby-catcher being a little too helpful; an excessive "welcome-to-my-world" slap between the shoulders.

During routine vaginal deliveries, the infant's head, neck, and shoulders bear the brunt of birthing, which can leave restrictions on critical structures such as nerves, arteries, the spinal cord, lungs, heart, and brain. Risks multiply when there are complications such as premature breaking of the amniotic sac, abnormal presentations, umbilical cord wrapped around the neck, aspiration of amniotic fluid, induced labor, forceps delivery, infections, internal bleeding, and so forth. For example, the instantaneous depressurization accompanying a C-Section allows the head to expand too rapidly, leaving strain patterns and restrictions in the skull, intracranial membranes, nerves, blood vessels, and brain. Likewise, forceps can crimp and damage the skull and underlying structures, dampen the motions of the cranial bones, and strain neck and shoulder tissues including arteries and nerves. Any of this can impede Central Nervous System (CNS) development.

The medulla oblongata (brain stem) is particularly vulnerable during birth and early in life because the musculature to support our head and protect our neck has not yet developed. Arguably the single most important structure in the CNS because it relays all nerve traffic in both directions between the brain and the rest of the body, the brainstem is also the origin of most of the cranial nerves, which control our special senses such as speech, sight, taste, smell, and hearing. The medulla is also the origin of another very important nerve, the vagus, which provides two-way communications between our brain and our thoracic and abdominal organs. Once the crisis has passed, this parasympathetic nerve calms those structures down and returns them to normal function when we've been under stress or in danger.

Birth trauma can impede the brain's arterial supply and drainage and Cerebrospinal Fluid (CSF) production, circulation, and reabsorption. This alone will affect the entire body. It may produce immediate symptoms, such as pain, rash, bruises, digestive problems such as colic, restlessness, and Sudden Infant Death Syndrome (SIDS) (crib death). Even absent immediate symptoms, however, birth trauma will surface eventually as challenges such as failure to thrive, cognitive and behavioral problems like ADD and ADHD, and chronic neck and shoulder tension. For example, while the aspiration of amniotic fluid from the birth canal is usually treated and quickly forgotten, the experience and resultant restrictions can eventually lead to decades of respiratory challenges, anxiety, panic attacks, and being stuck in fight-or-flight.

Given the relative novelty of manual therapy, it's not surprising that manual therapists routinely encounter patients who have been unknowingly carrying birth trauma for decades. The possibility of unrecognized birth trauma argues for early intervention and periodic follow up. Indeed, in osteopathic hospitals where newborns received manual therapy within hours or days of delivery, the incidence of birthing complications such as SIDS is dramatically reduced.

Adhesions

A common if largely overlooked restriction type, adhesions can proliferate very rapidly after surgery or internal bleeding and infections. These abnormal, fascial cobwebs occur after internal tissues have been exposed to air or gasses, even during arthroscopic procedures Their existence after a surgery does not suggest that there was something wrong with the procedure, however, they occasionally become so problematic that the doctor will feel compelled to surgically remove them. Manual therapy can break up adhesions, though it can be uncomfortable and time-consuming if the adhesions are large. A third option, the external applications of castor oil packs, while messy, is an effective and inexpensive way to dissolve adhesions and soften scar tissues. (For instructions, please see Appendix C: Castor Oil Packs.)

Emotional Content and Physical Trauma

Many restrictions are primarily emotional or have an emotional component. Because our bodies are hard-wired for survival, the nervous system automatically dumps "content" (emotions, issues, beliefs, judgments, and attitudes) into our bodies whenever we have an overload. In times of stress or physical or emotional danger, this dumping occurs instantaneously and without our conscious awareness. When the content lands in or around the site of an injury, infection, or surgery, it may delay or even stall recovery.

Content increases the likelihood and tenacity of restrictions and adhesions. Indeed, it can also create them. Therefore, whenever injuries or surgeries are slow to heal in otherwise-healthy individuals, emotional content may be in play and the possibility should be thoroughly explored. When emotional content creates or maintains a restriction, addressing the emotional component usually expedites the release and subsequent recovery. (Chapter 7, BodyMind explores this topic in depth.)

How the Body Responds to Force

When an external physical force interacts with the body, the body's first strategy is to let the associated energy dissipate. If the force exceeds the tissue's capacity for dissipation, however, the body's response is to concentrate the energy into as small an area as possible. This minimizes the effect on the entire organism, especially initially. Over time, however, this encapsulated energy acts like the proverbial grain of sand in the oyster's shell, forming a pathological pearl.

The mechanical energy associated with trauma tends to pass through less dense tissues and lodge in more dense structures like bones, blood vessels, and solid organs like the heart, liver, and spleen. Mechanical force also tends to follow the fascia, parallel to the long axis of the body and converge on joints and transiting structures such as blood vessels and nerves. For this reason, when a joint is painful or restricted, transiting structures should be checked because the body may have sacrificed joint movement and function to protect more important structures such as the heart or CNS.

Energy Cysts

Generally speaking, cysts are small packets of cells walled off from neighboring tissues. The force or energy associated with mechanical injuries disturbs the body's energy field. Dr. Upledger found that if the incoming energy exceeds the amount that the tissue can dissipate, the body will concentrate it into the smallest area possible. Having heard Dr. Upledger describe this, Dr. Elmer Green at the Menninger Foundation suggested that these concentrations sounded like energy cysts, a term Upledger readily accepted.

Quanta

The forces associated with impacts enter the body in straight lines. Relative to the force, however, the body is either already in motion or moves during the impact. In other words, the input direction and final destinations change continuously. Therefore, if we were to watch the interaction between incoming force and the body in very slow motion, we would see that rather than entering in a single linear dose, the force actually arrives in hundreds or thousands of discrete micro-doses, along an ever-changing series of straight lines. This process begins at the moment of impact and continues until the incoming force stops and the body comes to a complete rest. In this sense, a single physical trauma can produce a restriction composed of hundreds of individual units of force and produce multiple overlapping or contiguous energy cysts.

Vectors

In addition to a physical skeleton, we also have an energetic one. The two should align, sharing the same geometry and position. However, physical or emotional trauma can break our energetic skeleton or offset it from our physical skeleton. Dr. Upledger called these breaks and deviations "vectors." While differing from mechanical restrictions, broken or skewed vectors also disrupt the body's energy field and impair our health and vitality. Patients with multiple injuries, for example from a car wreck or sports, may have half a dozen or more broken vectors.

Trauma Quanta and Vectors

It may be tempting to dismiss talk of energy and energetic skeletons as something fanciful and unproven, however, this has been well-accepted for thousands of years in some parts of the world, like China. Furthermore, exciting new research suggests that the energetic skeleton or blueprint drives our development from conception to adulthood and beyond. Readers can learn more about this at the website www.thelivingmatrixmovie.com. The bottom line is that if there are breaks in the energetic skeleton, we'll feel much better and more unified when they're repaired.

CHAPTER 5

The Needle in the Haystack: How We Find Restrictions

Three factors conspire to hide restrictions and underscore the importance of manual skills. The first is our body's built-in ability to absorb trauma and compensate for restrictions. How could it be otherwise? We would never live to maturity if our design were One (trauma) and Done.

Time is the second factor: because of compensation and recruitment, years may pass before a given restriction begins to produce a detectable symptom. By then, we're likely to have forgotten the injury or illness or assumed it's no longer an issue.

Finally, traumas frequently lodge at a distance from the point of impact. For example, a blow on the left temple can produce a restriction diagonally across the head in the right occiput, or even in the neck. Or, when we bang the top of our head, some of the force may travel down our spine and lodge in our sacroiliac joints, jamming the sacrum bilaterally. Conversely, should we fall on our butt, some of the force may travel up the spine and lodge in the joint between our first cervical vertebra and our head. In fact, these cranium-sacrum patterns are very common.

A classic example of displaced force is the spleen. While the bulk of the impact from a shoulder strap, air bag, steering wheel, or car seat may have been initially absorbed by the sternum and ribs, the excess would reach the pericardium and heart. Composed largely of muscle, the heart is a relatively strong, flexible hollow organ that points downward and to the left. This orientation directs incoming force at the comparatively fragile spleen which has been known to rupture as long as eight weeks after a motor vehicle collision. Also in the line of fire is the left kidney which can rupture or end up stuck in a descended position. Both organs should be checked once the danger of rupture has passed.

Finding restrictions distant from the point of impact could be a challenge. However, CranioSacral and Visceral Manipulation are ideal for that. The next section describes several of their most common and effective techniques.

Cranial Rhythm as a Restriction Locator

Strongest in the cranium, the cranial rhythm should be detectable and symmetrical everywhere. Therefore, anomalies or distortions in the rhythm alert us to the presence of restrictions and help us pinpoint their location. For example, a strong cranial rhythm in both hips but only one thigh suggests there is a restriction in the thigh with the weaker rhythm. The restriction will be where the rhythm is first interrupted as we move toward the knee from the hip. Similarly, if the cranial rhythm on one side of the head is stronger than on the other, a restriction is impacting the weaker side and the cranial rhythm will help us find it.

"Arcing" Restrictions

As mentioned before, energy cysts actively disturb surrounding tissues and broadcast perceptible energetic ripples outward, in ever expanding, ever weakening circles, similar to what happens when we drop a pebble in a pool of water. Using both hands, we can pinpoint energy cysts by triangulation—the ripples will feel stronger to the hand that is closer. This process is called "arcing" because our hands are sensing a segment (or arc) of those circular ripples.

Manual therapists can arc passively or actively. Passive arcing entails simply receiving the energetic pulses with our hands. Active arcing involves sending energy from both hands and listening for the bounce or reflection from the cyst. This is like radar, similar to the way bats and marine mammals echolocate. Both approaches allow us to find energy cysts from anywhere on the body. Indeed, since the energetic disturbances continue out into space, some practitioners can arc from off-body, even from across the room.

Energy cysts often contain emotional content. Treatments resulting in the resurfacing and release of emotions are called SomatoEmotional Releases (SERs). We'll explore them more fully in Chapter 7.

Fascial Pull as Restriction Locator

Typically, mechanical restrictions attract our hands thanks to the elastic nature of fascia. We follow that attraction or pull until we've arrived directly over the restriction. If we then go neutral, we may sense something subtle. If our hand feels pulled into the body, the restriction is primarily physical. However, if the tissue gently repels our hand, the underlying restriction is more emotional. If the tissues on opposite sides of an incision pull into the scar, the restriction is primarily physical. However, if the tissues on both sides feel as if they are trying to separate, an emotion is involved. Typically, emotional content responds best to a lighter touch.

Fascial pulls can even lead us to restrictions in and under bones. For example, when we gently compress the frontal bone toward the occiput, if there is a restriction in the brain, the bones will move toward it and our hands will be pulled into it. If the patient's neck starts to relax and lengthen while we're doing this, the patient's primary restriction is almost certainly somewhere in the head. However, if the patient's neck tightens and shortens or if we feel a pull downward into the body, the restriction in the head is connected to a larger one in the body.

Similarly, a restriction inside the thorax will attract our hand when we gently press the sternum toward the spine. It could be on any number of structures: the mediastinum, pericardium, heart, artery, vein, lung, or one of the heart's three suspensory ligaments. Once, we've followed the pull all the way to where it stops, we'll have a pretty good idea which structure it's on.

Vectors

Therapists who can see the energetic skeleton are also able to see breaks or offsets in it. Even those who don't see vectors can often feel that something is amiss, which is the first step in correcting the problem.

Visceral Mobility and Motilities as Restriction Locators

Lack of either visceral mobility or motility indicates the presence of restrictions. Restrictions on thoracic and abdominal viscera are often visually noticeable if they interfere with the expansion of the thorax with each inhalation. Asymmetries in the motility of internal organs point directly to restrictions. When there are multiple restrictions, an organ will move most strongly toward the strongest one acting upon it.

Thermal Projections

Whenever there is pathology in a tissue, there will be a thermal projection off the body directly over it. We can use our hands to find these projections. They mimic the shape of the structure involved, helping us determine exactly where the restriction is. Readers can learn more about all of this in Dr. Barral's *Manual Thermal Diagnosis*.

Dr. Barral's research shows that the human hand can detect thermal anomalies as slight as 4/1000th of a degree centigrade. This acuity has enabled Dr. Barral to find tumors that MRIs have missed. While exceptional, Dr. Barral's sensitivity underscores the sophistication, precision, and power of the human hand and partially accounts for its therapeutic potential. Most manual listening skills are teachable, though practitioners will gravitate toward those techniques best suited to their individual gifts and personal preferences.

Energetic Shells

This may come as a surprise but, like Russian dolls, numerous energetic shells surround the body. I would remind skeptics that just because we are unaware of something or don't see it doesn't mean that it's not there, is unimportant, or doesn't affect us. Gravity is an obvious example. In any event, there may be a dozen or more of these envelopes extending many feet out from our body, with names like spiritual, etheric, mental, astral, soul, akashic, and so forth. While manual therapists typically focus on the physical, emotional, and spiritual envelopes, we are undoubtedly affecting others at times.

The physical shell is on the body. The emotional envelope is the first off the body, three or four inches out, followed by the spiritual, ten to twelve inches out. We sometimes dismiss emotional upsets by saying, "it's just emotional," suggesting that our feelings are of little consequence. Then we may laugh, suggesting that we know better and that stuffing or denying these upsets doesn't work very well and is a recipe for depression and other problems.

Given the current preoccupation with the physical and material, our discounting the import of our feelings is understandable, if mistaken. Likewise, we can be forgiven for assuming that a leak in the physical shell has more health significance than one in the emotional or spiritual shell. However, Dr. Barral and other experts believe that leaks in the emotional envelope are more serious than in the physical because they drain us energetically and leave us more vulnerable to illness and injury. Furthermore, according to these same experts, leaks in the spiritual envelope are even more serious as they entail the loss of more energy more quickly than leaks in the emotional shell.

(Chapter 10 explores the distinction between emotional and spiritual content, but the primary difference is that spiritual content typically affects our relationship with ourselves, which is more serious than our feelings.) Interestingly, when patients find spiritual content in their tissues, they usually sit up and take notice, even if they normally don't give a moment's thought to spiritual matters and regardless of their religious beliefs or inclinations. Indeed, their responses seem to suggest that they instinctively recognize the importance of spiritual content.

Lesional Chains

Previously, we mentioned that traumas lodge in denser tissues and that restrictions render tissues denser than normal. Therefore, it should be no surprise that restrictions attract subsequent traumas as if there were a beaten path to it—which, in a sense, there is. These paths are particularly perceptible in the case of penetration wounds from stabbing, bullets, arrows, spears, and the like.

Another perceptible path involves two or more restrictions that have somehow become mechanically connected. Recognizing these lesional chains is important because unless all the elements are treated at the same time as a single system, the chain tends to persist. Indeed, the reappearance of a treated restriction may be a clue that we failed to detect a chain. Eliminating the elements of the chain and the connecting paths also reduces the likelihood of re-injury.

With chains, the fascia usually pulls toward one of the restrictions. For example, while treating a patient's head, we felt a fascial pull down into her heart. From there, we were immediately drawn further down the midline along a caesarian scar to a hysterectomy scar above her pubic bone. From there, the pull veered to the right, before finally stopping at an appendectomy scar from childhood. This chain included emotional trauma from physical abuse. By releasing the emotional trauma and lining up all the scars and tensions from her head to her appendectomy, we disrupted this chain, significantly reducing the frequency and intensity of her migraines and headaches. This segues nicely into our next topic, treatment.

CHAPTER 6

Out! Out! Release Techniques

Some restrictions release the instant they are found, thereby muddying the distinction between finding and treating. For the purposes of discussion, however, we've separated finding and treating into distinct chapters. Most manual therapy treatment techniques fall into one of four broad categories: direction of ease, traction, direction of energy, or some combination thereof. All involve the intention that whatever is in the patient's best interest will occur. If a restriction does not release, we can explore why, we can try all of our tricks, but ultimately, the choice is the patient's.

Direction of Ease

As the name suggests, this category involves following and even encouraging the tissue to go where it prefers; usually this is into the restriction. Direction of ease is osteopathic in the sense that it aligns with the tissue's natural tendencies. Usable on any tissue, the most common direction of ease techniques include approximation, recoil, and unwindings.

Approximation

Approximation involves following fascial tension into the restriction and then backing off ever so slightly, allowing subsequent movements, and then following them using more approximation until the tensions line up precisely in all three planes, whereupon the restriction usually releases.

CranioSacral Therapy (CST) uses approximation on cross-body diaphragms, joints, cranial sutures (the joints between the bones of the head), and vectors. For example, if two cranial bones are jammed together because of a restriction on the joint, we can often gain a release by encouraging the two bones to move even closer. This mimics the technique for opening a sticky drawer: closing it and trying again. Similarly, we open cabinets with magnetic closures by pushing the magnets closer together until they repel each other, then we release the pressure, thereby allowing the door to pop open.

Approximation also works wonders on joints that have been injured by jamming, torquing, and overuse. The resultant misalignment can eventually destroy the joint's articular surfaces, necessitating replacement surgery. Gently supporting and following the bones into the restriction allows them to realign and redistributes the fluid that lubricates and cushions the joint surfaces. Try this should you jam a finger or other digit or sprain an ankle or wrist.

Another place where approximation works miracles is in the paired long bones of the lower leg or lower arm. In the lower leg for example, the tibia and fibula work in concert with each other, allowing us to turn our foot inward and outward and invert and evert our ankle. Similarly, the radius and ulna of the lower arm dance around each other, allowing us to rotate our hands from palm down (pronation) to palm up (supination).

As if they'd been wound too tightly around each other, a pair will often realign and rebalance themselves when we gently squeeze together their distal ends (just above the ankle or wrist). This approximation releases the tensional imbalances in the membrane between them, improving range of motion and function to the joints directly above (elbow and knee) and below (ankle and wrist). While the technique is essentially mechanical, feeling the bones choreograph their own realignment and the joints opening has a hydraulic quality and can be delightful for practitioner and patient alike.

Vectors

Approximation also works wonders on vectors, those breaks in the energetic skeleton. We align the broken structure and then allow the two ends to move toward each other, much as a surgeon would with an offset fracture. Then we can move the energetic skeleton to the physical skeleton or vice versa until the two are aligned and restored to their ideal configuration. The process is analogous to clicking and dragging with the cursor to move text or symbols on a computer screen. These quick and painless techniques leave patients feeling a new sense of ease and integration.

Recoil

When approximation fails to win the day, we can add recoil, which takes advantage of the cyclical increase in tissue tensions associated with our breathing. Icing on the approximation cake, recoils consist of following the tissues as far as they take us and then popping our hands off very rapidly at the instant inhalation begins. Like sneaking up on someone who is carrying a dinner tray and saying "Boo!" recoils startle the tissues into abandoning old holding patterns. They are especially effective on lung restrictions where the explosive force associated with the onset of inhalation are the strongest of anywhere in the body and can be used to greatest advantage. While recoils may sound shocking, even violent, they aren't. Instead, they usually produce a sense of relaxation, lightness, expansion, spaciousness, and pleasant tingling. Even when patients are surprised almost out of their skin, they usually end up chuckling or laughing.

Recoils are also effective for releasing restrictions in bones. While we tend to think of bones as solid even rigid, they are anything but. A restricted bone can entrain overlying muscles and tissues. The resultant fascial tensions alert us to the existence of underlying restrictions. These entrainments may be visible, even to casual observers, especially in flat bones. For example, we occasionally see sternums so inwardly dished that they look like they could hold half a cup of liquid if their owners were lying on their backs.

As previously mentioned, living bone is plastic, continuously adapting to the forces acting upon it. With restrictions in bones, we encourage both ends of the bone into the restriction using direction-of-ease. We compress gently, so that the bone will lead us into its strain pattern. With bones the timing differs: We recoil, not at the moment inhalation begins, but at the point in the breath cycle where tensions in the bone are at maximum.

Unwinding/Regional Tissue Release

In therapeutic settings, when the body returns to the position it was in at the moment of impact, the stored energy may release spontaneously. Thanks to the repositioning, those linear avenues along which the mechanical energy entered can now serve as exit paths for that energy. It's analogous to changing the direction of traffic lanes to accommodate rush hour into and out of the city. We call this technique either "regional tissue release" which focuses on the effect, or "unwinding," which describes the process' appearance.

Fortunately, the therapist needn't try to locate all these "therapeutic" positions, as doing so might verge on the impossible. Instead, assuming the therapist is sufficiently light-handed and willing to surrender the reins, the patient's body wisdom choreographs the release, visiting all the necessary positions in the optimal sequence.

Regardless of whether the movements are large and dramatic or small and subtle, the therapist remains passive, supporting the unwinding structures just enough to neutralize the effect of gravity without inhibiting the movements. The energy stored in the patient's tissues powers the release. Waves of heat or energy emanating from the injured area are a common sign of release.

Patients who've just experienced dramatic unwindings may be tempted to imbue the therapist with supernatural powers; however, unwindings actually demonstrate the opposite, namely that the power and wisdom comes from the patient's body, not the practitioner. Indeed, unwindings remind us that even the most gifted manual therapists are merely facilitators, not healers.

Hear No Evil, See No Evil, Speak No Evil

Nearing the end of a treatment, I was drawn to the left side of a patient's head. As he lay on his back, face up on the massage table, my hands were drawn to the joint between his left temporal bone and his occiput. Before I could find the restriction, his head began to push backward, downward, into the massage table—a common sign of a neck ready to unwind.

Supporting his head and neck, I had him scoot part-way off the table until the table's edge caught the middle of his shoulder blades and the table would not interfere with his neck's unwinding. Though I'd facilitated some dramatic unwindings in my career, I was wholly unprepared for what happened next: his head and neck continued to push backwards toward the floor. (There was no stopping this one.) In order to cancel out the effects of gravity without interfering with the unwinding, I had to keep moving my hands.

Eventually, he was facing the floor while still on his back, his neck extended backwards 140 degrees. Normally, most of us can only extend our head back about 60 degrees. I could never have put his head in such an extreme position. Had I tried, I would have broken his neck long before his head reached 90 degrees, paralyzing or killing him. However, his body wisdom knew exactly what it needed to do. (I'm guessing that somehow, his bones and connective tissues had temporarily reverted to their childhood plasticity and elasticity.)

Within seconds, he said, "I see the carpet on the stairs in the house I grew up in. I'm about two. My mom is holding me. She's screaming into my left ear, 'I hate you! I hate you! I hate you!' Wow! Maybe that's why I've never been able hear out of that ear? She pitches me headfirst down the stairs. I land on the top of my head. Must've almost broken my neck."

I supported his head while waves of heat released from his shoulders, neck, and the back of his head. My patient shed a few tears. After several minutes, his head gradually began returning to a more normal position. Once he was face up, his head and neck waggled gently in progressively smaller arcs for another minute or two, as is common toward the end of neck unwindings. When it was completely finished, I helped him scoot back on the table. We released the restriction between his left temporal bone and occiput and balanced him out. I helped him off the table, offered him water, and encouraged him to drink as much water as he could in the next few hours. Once he felt grounded, he went on his way.

Research in neuroplasticity shows that when traumatic experiences resurface in therapeutic settings the brain reprocesses them and generates new neural pathways so that the associated content no longer keeps us in fight-or-flight. Since this unwinding had arisen unbidden and was unstoppable once it began, there was no doubt that he'd been ready for it. I'd just happened along at the right time.

Even so, I called him that evening to make sure he was okay. He said that he felt surprisingly well, considering, but was hearing static in his left ear. He asked if this was normal. I suggested that it sounded like his hearing might be coming back but after 35 years off-line, it might take his brain a little time to make sense of the input. (The next evening, he called to say he was hearing out of his left ear.)

Don't be misled by the above example. Unwindings are rarely that dramatic, physically or emotionally. They don't necessarily involve the overt release of content. But when powerful memories or feelings arise, it's because on some unconscious level the patient is ready and feels safe. While there are other ways to release trauma and restrictions from the body, none are so visible as unwindings.

Loss of Control

Unwindings are analogous to what a spring does when releasing its stored energy. Because we are unaccustomed to our body behaving as if it had a mind of its own, it may be tempting to assume that the manual therapist must be driving the movement. I've experienced osteopaths imposing an unwinding, but it feels completely different. Spontaneous unwindings usually feel wonderful. However, this too can be confusing, especially for those not accustomed to feeling wonderful or whose default way of being is to stay numb. Therefore, unwindings occasionally confuse the senses, leaving us feeling disoriented, anxious, fearful, or even angry. Those feelings may not be new, either, but part of the original injury. Often, the confusion stems from the fact that the body does not distinguish between past, present, and future.

Occasionally, a patient will dismiss an unwinding as hocus pocus or "woo-woo." Uncomfortable with the idea that their mind is not in control, they deal with the accompanying disorientation and fear by projecting imagined paranormality onto the therapist. Ironically, the patient's bodymind was in control the entire time. Of course, this can be a huge threat to the ego, which values control over everything, including our health and even life.

Patients who believe that the body is impure and therefore must be kept in check continually may feel threatened when theirs spontaneously unwinds. Unwindings may be unusual, but they are normal, natural, and healthy. In the majority of cases, any lack of ease with the process stems from its novelty. To me, unwindings are the Inner Physician or body wisdom made visible, a manifestation of the divine within us.

Traction

In many ways the antithesis of all the direction-of-ease techniques, traction involves gently engaging the fascia and waiting for the collagen to respond. Think of it as ironing or stretching out the fascial kinks and wrinkles and restoring normal linearity, plasticity, elasticity, and compensatory ability to muscles, tendons, ligaments, bones, blood vessels, nerves, and internal organs.

Therapeutic traction is gentle, not forceful. It's not a tug of war, contest of wills, or imposition of some preconceived notion on the tissues, but an invitation to the tissue to change. In fact, traction works best when, once a restriction is engaged, we back off enough to allow the tissue to subtly choreograph the release. Direct, relentless, overpowering stretches are no substitute for therapeutic manual traction. Living tissues rarely release in straight lines, which explains the limitations of mechanical traction devices.

Indeed, without ever completely abandoning gentle traction, manual therapists often find themselves dancing between direction-of-ease and traction, varying their techniques from moment to moment as their experience, intuition, felt sense, and the patient's tissues dictate. Such releases balance the therapist's traction and intention with the tissues' needs from moment to moment, whether it's unwinding, traction, and approximation, or something else.

We often combine approximation and unwinding when treating the joints between the bones of the head. First, we address the osseous restrictions (between the bones), using direction-of-ease, direction-of-energy, and traction. Then, using the bones for handles, we engage the membranous restrictions, again with gentle traction and direction of ease and energy. We listen, follow, and use intention as necessary, while maintaining our slightest traction.

Direction-of-Energy

Therapists can direct energy into restrictions, using hands and intention. To be clear, the energy directed is not the therapist's, but universal energy which is free, unlimited, and untainted. We don't use our own energy, because our energy does not belong in someone else's body, and vice versa. Using the mind, visualization, or their own hands, any person can direct this universal energy (sometimes called Reiki) into their own restrictions at any time.

The fact that many restrictions release the moment the patient gives himself permission to heal suggests that healing is mostly about the mind and permission. If a restriction doesn't release on its own, the patient can help by breathing into the area, allowing the area to soften, visualizing letting the restriction go, or visualizing energy flowing into the area.

People who are products of western cultures tend to participate actively in their therapy by doing something, anything. There's nothing wrong with this. It communicates willingness and intention to the tissues. After all, healing is not a spectator sport. Therefore, I often encourage these patients to visualize letting go of the restriction and exhaling any associated content. If a patient believes it would be helpful, I encourage them to replace afflictive content such as hate, anger, or fear with something positive such as self-compassion, self-love, self-forgiveness, peace, or acceptance.

You Are So Busted!

If the restriction is held in place by content or contains buried content, the mere discovery of this content may be enough to occasion the release. (We'll explore content and its release in the next chapter.) Since the process by which feelings and beliefs end up in tissues is instantaneous and unconscious, it shouldn't be surprising that the release of the content may be too. Often, the therapist feels the tissues change the instant that the patient begins remembering the content or thinking about letting it go. Faster-than-the-speed-of-thought comes to mind but in reality, such changes are merely faster than the speed of the thoughts' articulation. However, the speed and spontaneity do strongly suggest that much of the content that we've unconsciously parked in our body no longer has any intrinsic significance.

Most patients are willing to let go of the content we find in their tissue. When there is reluctance, it usually stems either from the novelty of the process or uncertainty about the consequences, especially if the content originated with some other person. A little education generally allays concerns. Failing that, we try to negotiate a win-win resolution. Chapter 11 explores the topic of resistance in depth.

Talking to Tissues

Dr. Upledger discovered by accident that it was possible to talk to tissues directly. While treating a restriction deep in his patient's brain, he suspected he might be working on the hypothalamus. He asked the structure what it did. Speaking through the patient's mouth, but in a gruff tone very different from the patient's normal voice, the tissue described functions typical of a hypothalamus. (The inflection (gruff voice) was also Upledger's first clue that some CNS structures might have their own personalities, distinct from other structures' or the patient's). When Upledger asked the structure if it was the hypothalamus, the structure confirmed that it was. A few days later, Upledger had a similar experience with a different CNS structure on a different patient.

Dr. Upledger had a knack for balancing healthy skepticism gained from his medical training with humility and open-mindedness learned from experience. This combination led him to a number of profound discoveries with therapeutic significance. In this case, he realized that he'd stumbled on a simple and effective protocol for optimizing brain structures. As he and his colleagues explored this protocol, the structures they engaged revealed that they performed psychological and emotional functions that neurologists had not previously considered. Thanks to Dr. Upledger and his colleagues, we have a pretty good idea what anatomical structure might be involved in a given issue, such as an inability to trust. Furthermore, being able to dialogue with the brain eliminates a great deal of guesswork and dramatically increases the amount of therapy one can accomplish in a given amount of time.

What's Good for the Goose...

As a patient, I've personally benefitted from being able to talk directly with the brain's structures. On one occasion, in response to a colleague's question, my brain reported that its blood supply was inadequate. The colleague traced the problem to a restriction in my left vertebral artery. (This situation is surprisingly common, owing to heaviness of the head and vulnerability of the neck's arteries.) My restriction stemmed from at least two whiplashes, one in infancy and the other when I was 36. Restoring adequacy required only about ten minutes, boosted Cerebrospinal Fluid (CSF) production and circulation, and allowed my entire body to relax.

From talking to brain components, it was a simple step to realize that it was possible to talk to any tissue in the body, provided a willing patient. As crazy as this may sound, it shouldn't be that surprising, given how smart our tissues are and how powerful the mind is. For example, Dr. Upledger discovered that he could talk directly to the immune system through the thymus, a small gland between our sternum and heart. Working with thymus makes it possible to eliminate adhesions and scar tissue, remove toxins and pharmaceutical residues, restore damaged tissues and organs to their former splendor, and even defuse dangerous feelings like rage. (This versatility and power are why Chapter 1 presents the thymus as an exemplar of the body's innate brilliance.) Working with thymus also makes it possible to eliminate allergies and treat a host of otherwise problematic immune and autoimmune challenges.

Here's where it gets very interesting: when all else fails, it's often possible to talk directly to mysterious and troubling symptoms. This can be extremely helpful. For example, I've had luck talking to chronic sinusitis and plantar fasciitis. Pain and other symptoms can be our body's way of getting our attention. Once the body has our attention and we understand what the problem is, we're positioned to make new, healthier choices. When a patient has a belief or theory about what's causing the problem, we can start there. Talking to symptoms can avoid exploring possibilities that prove to be dead ends.

Help from on High

We can also enlist the help of the Inner Physician, that wise part of us that knows what's best for us and how to heal. We can also enlist the centrum, another "structure" in the loosest sense of the word that Dr. Upledger and his colleagues discovered. Our direct, personal connection to the divine, centrum is an almost impeccable source of insight and guidance because it knows our unique spiritual path. (For a full discussion of centrum, see Chapter 9.)

Adhesions Be Gone

We can use traction to free up tissues from the effects of adhesions, but working with large ones can be time-consuming and uncomfortable for the patient. While the immune system is capable of eliminating adhesions, my personal bias is to save it for freeing up adhesions and restrictions on critical structures like blood vessels, nerves, the brain, internal organs, and extremely toxic and dangerous emotions. My rationale is that the immune system is busy enough, in general, keeping us safe from pathogens, and so forth. Therefore, if someone has massive adhesions or scars, I normally encourage them to invest their own time and energy doing castor oil packs. Applied externally, these wool flannel packs will dissolve adhesions and soften scar tissues, even the massive ones that sometimes follow abdominal surgery and major trauma. (See Appendix C for instructions.)

The immune system will be involved in cleaning up the debris and repairing and replacing any damaged tissue, but asking it to take the lead on something we can accomplish ourselves with a castor oil pack strikes me as a waste of a powerful resource we may need for something more important soon.

Elevated RAS

The Reticular Activating System (RAS) is the part of the CNS that focuses on our safety and survival. Unfortunately, like a faulty gauge, the RAS can get stuck in the elevated alert mode known as fight-or-flight. Actually, because it includes two less exercised options, it would be more accurate to call the condition "fight, flight, freeze, or fold" but as that would be too cumbersome, for convenience we talk as if there were only the two.

Usually, RAS gets stuck when we've been exposed to stress or danger that we weren't able to fight or flee from. These situations are exceedingly common, much more so than most of us realize. They include being bullied, harassed, criticized, blamed, shamed, given impossible tasks, or endangered during infancy, childhood, and when we're adults. It can happen at home, at school, in sports, in play, or at work. Elevated RAS can even occur *in utero* if mom is in danger or otherwise endangering us. Though largely unrecognized, elevated RASs are exceedingly common, even in relatively safe nations like the US, and constitute an unrecognized pandemic with global implications for health and safety.

From the tissue's perspective, elevated RAS is not so much a mechanical restriction as a functional challenge. While less problematic than Post-Traumatic Stress Disorder (PTSD), having an elevated RAS negatively affects the entire body. Symptoms include chronically tight muscles and digestive, immune, endocrine, cognitive, attention, and sleep challenges.

Most patients and their doctors will not connect these symptoms to being stuck in fight-or-flight, largely because it never occurs to either party that that might be what's going on. However, finding out is a simple matter. We just ask the body directly where RAS is set on a scale of 1-100. Numerical answers such as 34 or 86 should be a good indication of how things stand, but qualitative answers such as fine, high, maxed out also suffice.

RAS resets are simple. We ask if one would be in the patient's best interest. If yes, then we ask what setting on that same 1-100 scale would be ideal in the immediate future. Given that information, we ask the body to reset the patient's RAS to whatever level is most appropriate. That's usually all it takes. Occasionally, we may have to revisit the issue to complete the reset or lower it even further if the patient realizes later that he or she would be even better off if the system was reset even lower.

Testimonial

In a workshop more than a decade ago, my body reported to the colleague practicing on me that my RAS was set at 80 on the 1-100 scale. I wasn't all that surprised. I'm guessing that I'd been stuck in fight-or-flight since infancy. The knowledge that it had been stuck helped explain certain past choices. Resetting my RAS required less than ten minutes and relaxed my entire body.

ACEs

In the last decade, medicine has grudgingly recognized Adverse Childhood Experiences (ACEs). A condition similar to RAS, ACEs contributes to academic challenges from primary school onward. It also produces adolescent truancy, drug and alcohol abuse, and criminal behavior and serious health challenges by the time people reach their 30s. ACEs tend to cluster in socioeconomically-stressed neighborhoods. However, my experience suggests that when they start looking, professionals will eventually find ACEs in children from affluent areas, too. The film "Resilience" is a great introduction to the syndrome and successful treatment strategies. To my knowledge, there have been no studies endeavoring to distinguish elevated RASs from ACEs.

The Philosophy of Allowance

With the body, it's important to remember that force rarely solves problems. Therefore, manual therapists do not "destroy the village to save it." One of Dr. Upledger's favorite mantras was "five grams of force and five million pounds of intention." Again, the intention is to accomplish whatever is in the patient's best interest. Only the patient and his body can know what that is. The manual therapist has to trust that whatever needs to happen will happen. If a restriction will not let go, there is probably a good reason. We have to respect that. It's not the manual therapist's job to judge or choose for the patient. We create safety and offer tools and options.

Physician, Heal Thyself

But more good news: the foregoing suggests that patients can release some of their restrictions without any help. That's how powerful the mind and the body's innate ability to heal are, separately or combined. A manual therapist should be able to help patients get started. (Chapter 15 explains how to find one.)

When it comes to treating restrictions, the body could care less where a technique comes from or what it is called. It's all about results, gently earned. Now that we've learned about how to find and release mechanical restrictions, we're ready to learn about how emotions and other content land in our tissues and how to release them, the subjects of the next three chapters.

CHAPTER 7

History of the BodyMind

Body and mind have always been inextricably connected. Traditional cultures have always known it, and our language reflects this inseparability. We ignore the connection at our own risk. Working with it enables us to overcome illness, heal injuries, and restore and optimize health, often without drugs, invasive procedures, and expensive technology.

Nothing New under the Sun

The growing consensus that body and mind are inseparable is hailed by some as a recent breakthrough and dismissed by others as New Age or "woo-woo." Both views are mistaken. There is nothing new, New Age, or weird about the body-mind connection. It is as old as history. Recent advances in neuroscience have shown that it is both real and hard-wired.

Indeed, if anything is novel, it's the misconception that body and mind are separate. Begun by the French philosopher René Descartes in the 17th Century, this notion reached its zenith in the first half of the 20th Century thanks to huge advances in medical technology. These encouraged people to view the body as a machine, illness as a malfunction that could be repaired with drugs and surgery, and injuries as just a matter of physics.

History is against those who believe that body and mind are separate. For example, as a formal practice, Traditional Chinese Medicine (TCM) has existed for 2500 years and has helped billions of people stay healthy and recover from illness. Indeed, the World Health Organization has deemed it effective for the treatment of more than 80 diseases. This effectiveness stems in part from TCM's viewing mind and body as inseparable. TCM recognizes 12 organ meridians, each associated with specific emotions, energies, attitudes, and tendencies. In other words, in TCM, mental, emotional, and physical health are closely linked. A challenge in one aspect usually implies a challenge in the other. More importantly, TCM uses this connection to guide us toward health in body, mind, and spirit.

For example, in TCM, when the kidneys are balanced energetically, a person will exhibit resolution, willpower, and trust in the presence of a challenge and apprehension and fear in the presence of danger. If the energy in the kidney meridian is deficient, however, the same or even a lesser challenge may produce timidity, inferiority, shame, fearfulness, panic, or phobia. If the energy in the kidney meridian is excessive, the same threat is more likely to engender audacity, foolhardiness, superiority, shamelessness, mistrust, suspiciousness, or paranoia.

Ayurveda, the 5,000-year-old medicine of India, also recognizes the connection between the emotions and health. Greek, Roman, and other Western cultures viewed the body and the mind as a unity in which the mind was as healthy as the body, and the body as healthy as the mind. In Latin, that would be *mens sana in corpore sano.*

Indeed, even the English language acknowledges the inseparability of physical, emotional, and spiritual health. For example, the word "disease" suggests that someone is "not at ease"—and not necessarily because they are sick. Indeed, it's just as likely that their "lack of ease" (stress) is why they became sick in the first place, as we will learn.

The words courage, encourage, discourage, and rancor all derive from the French word for heart, *coeur*. We speak of efforts that are whole-hearted or half-hearted. A person wishes he could be more supportive, but his heart isn't in it. A person wants to end a relationship, but she hasn't the heart, either because she has no stomach for conflict or hopes to avoid hurting the other person's feelings. People are said to be sick at heart and broken-hearted. Indeed, heartbroken people sometimes die from their inability to withstand the loss of a companion, mate, family member, friend, or pet.

We vent our spleen. We're full of bile. Cheeky people are said to have a lot of gall. Really angry people are livid. We have the crap and pee scared or beaten out of us. Spineless people do not lack anatomical backbones; instead, they can't stand up for themselves, or for others, or for their convictions. These expressions are more than figures of speech. They stem from centuries of observation and experience.

Given the English language's reputation for precision, it seems ironic that English has no single word for the unity between body, mind, emotion, and spirit. However, in the last 50 years, to express this essential unity, the term "bodymind" has come into use and is now found in Reichian psychology, Asian bodywork, and psychoneuroimmunology, the new science studying the relationship between the mind and the nervous and immune systems. While most healing arts practitioners take the relationship as a given, much of what we understand about how this unity actually works stems from quantum advances in imaging technology, microbiology, biochemistry, and neuroscience.

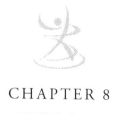

CHAPTER 8

Somatomization and Communication: How the BodyMind Works

To function as a unit, body and mind must be in constant communication. They are, thanks to the nervous system (and the fascia, as explained in Chapter 2). There are so many different aspects of the nervous system—for example, central, peripheral, sympathetic, parasympathetic—that the terminology can get a little confusing. All we really need to know for the present discussion is that there are afferent and efferent nerves. Afferent nerves carry information to the (Central Nervous System/CNS) and are also called sensory nerves because they tell the brain what's going on out in the tissues. Efferent nerves carry impulses from the CNS and brain and are often called motor nerves because they tell the tissues, whether it's a muscle or an internal organ, what to do. Together, the afferent and efferent nerves make this two-way communication possible. Occasionally, a single nerve or set of nerves carries information in both directions. In Chapter 4, we mentioned the vagus, Cranial Nerve X, as a prime example of a bi-directional nerve.

Somatomization

Somatomization is a technical term commonly used in manual therapy to describe the normal process of moving content out of our mind into our soma (tissues). Content includes emotions and feelings, thoughts, ideas, issues, beliefs, attitudes, agreements, understandings, pledges, and oaths.

Somatomization should not be confused with somatization, a term which medicine until recently defined as a mental disorder in which the subject has numerous physical complaints that cannot be explained by any medical condition or as an effect of chemicals. But these complaints are not seen as intentionally manufactured by the subject. Somatization has recently been renamed somatic symptom disorder (SSD) and is defined in the DSM-V as "a person having a significant focus on physical symptoms, such as pain, weakness or shortness of breath, that results in major distress and/or problems functioning. The individual has excessive thoughts, feelings and behaviors relating to the physical symptoms. The physical symptoms may or may not be associated with a diagnosed medical condition, but the person is experiencing symptoms and believes they are sick (that is, not faking the illness)."

Whether somatization is an actual mental problem or a misdiagnosis of unusually physically sensitive people remains to be seen. However, somatomization is not a mental illness, but a normal, healthy frequently used neurological reflex. It occurs automatically, unconsciously, and instantaneously when something exceeds our ability to deal with it in the moment. Designed for our survival, it allows us to ignore distractions and focus on the task at hand whether the latter is something mundane like finishing our homework, doing the dishes, or playing sports, or something critical like driving through a blizzard or wildfire or escaping from a burning building. In addition to allowing us to live so that we can fight another day, dumping content into tissues can also help maintain our sanity and ability to function in otherwise overwhelming conditions.

What constitutes an overload depends on our situation: namely, how busy, safe, healthy, and physically and emotionally strong we are. Stress, responsibilities, preoccupations, danger, injuries, illness, setbacks, and surgery often render us more vulnerable to overload, and therefore more likely to park content in our tissues. In other words, we might be able to deal with and process a given input on nine days out of ten; however, on that tenth day, when we are under the weather, under pressure, or in danger, that same input might exceed our processing capacity. When this happens, our nervous system instantly dumps that input somewhere in our body without our awareness. And there it stays.

No Free Lunch

The primary avenues of somatomization are the sympathetic nerves of the autonomic nervous system. As the word *autonomic* suggests, these nerves are largely beyond conscious control; in other words, they are autonomous and automatic. As sophisticated as humans and our bodies may be, the CNS apparently has not learned to distinguish physical threats from psychological or emotional threats and treats all the same. When we experience an overload, the sympathetic nervous system dumps the overload in our tissues while mobilizing us for fight-or-flight by raising our blood pressure, blood sugar, and blood oxygen levels and flooding our body with stress hormones like cortisol and adrenalin.

While helping us survive in the short term, parked content can create mechanical restrictions and hold pre-existing ones in place. Although we don't know the content is there, it communicates continuously with the amygdala thanks to those afferent nerves. The part of our brain that processes emotions, the amygdala concludes that we are in physical danger because it does not readily distinguish between past threats that have been stored in our tissues and current threats. This explains why people who suffer from PTSD sometimes suddenly find themselves reliving the original trauma.

In any event, this communication leaves us stuck in fight-or-flight, which has significant health consequences. We touched on this in the discussion of RAS at the end of Chapter 5. For starters, our immune and digestive systems are put on hold. Our heart works harder. Our adrenal glands leak adrenalin, and we run the risk of adrenal fatigue and exhaustion. We don't sleep as deeply as we need. Our thinking may be compromised because the CNS may divert some of the arterial blood normally destined for the cerebral cortex to the structures that orchestrate survival.

Ironically, in addition to impairing our health, being stuck in fight-or-flight also leaves us less safe. For starters, it impedes our ability to detect actual danger because the part of the CNS responsible, the Reticular Activating System (RAS), is already overloaded. Consisting mainly of the pons, medulla oblongata, cerebellum, and amygdala, the reticular structures (or formation) are designed to handle about 100 million neural impulses per second. When we are stuck in fight-or-flight, however, they attempt to monitor all our neurological traffic, about 5.1 billion impulses per second, approximately 50 times their capacity.

Our ability to run or fight in response to danger will also be impaired because our muscles are already partially contracted, and we've been leaking rather than storing adrenalin, which is essentially our body's rocket-fuel. In other words, while somatomization can save our lives and safeguard our emotional and mental health in the moment, it entails significant long-term costs. Fortunately, there are simple techniques that enable the CNS to process and release this somatomized content and the associated restrictions.

It's Just Stress

Somatomized content also significantly diminishes our ability to manage stress. Stress occurs whenever we perceive, consciously or otherwise, that current or imminent demands exceed our capabilities. The medical effects of stress are well known. They include ulcers and other digestive challenges, hypertension, heart disease, weight gain, adrenal fatigue and exhaustion, and so forth. The American Medical Association estimates that 80% of illness is stress related, which is why stress is often called "the silent killer."

Some physicians call our gut "the second brain" to underscore its neurological importance. The constant communication between our gut and our CNS means that digestive challenges tend to keep us in fight-or-flight, adding to our stress. The gall bladder is a favorite repository for stress, which explains why 350,000 gall bladders are surgically removed in America each year. (The gall bladder stores bile, which is essential for digesting fats. If you are challenged digesting fats or have a history of gallstones, your gall bladder may be at risk.) While these surgeries may be medically necessary, removing the gall bladder doesn't address the cause if it is stress.

Indeed, losing our gall bladder can add to our stress because it leaves us unable to digest fats—an important food category, forces dietary changes, and complicates dining out and with others. Furthermore, with the gall bladder gone, stress now focuses on the stomach, producing ulcers and other digestive challenges. Therefore, at the first sign of gall bladder challenges, we should be evaluating our stress level, finding ways to reduce it, and exploring proven stress management techniques such as physical and energy exercises, mindfulness, meditation, knitting, gardening, fishing, painting—whatever works for us.

Stress Reflex

While studying and publicizing the biochemistry of stress, medicine has largely ignored its mechanical effects, even though the two are intimately related and the mechanical is at least as significant. Thanks to another reflex, stress tightens our respiratory diaphragm. This significantly reduces the amount of air we can inhale. The tension also impacts structures connected to and passing through the diaphragm. The former includes the spine, liver, stomach, spleen, lungs, heart, pericardium, and thymus gland. The latter includes the abdominal aorta, portal vein, inferior vena cava, esophagus, various nerve ganglions and plexi (crossroads), and important lymphatic ducts.

The stress reflex is often readily apparent in small children who haven't learned how to hide it. Most of us either had one or more of those meltdowns when we were young, or have seen similar at the grocery store or airport. Adults are more adept at concealing their stress, but that doesn't make it any less impactful on their health.

Insurmountable

In contemplating the ripple effects of stress, it's helpful to remember that fascia connects every cell in the body and, therefore, can have dramatic and immediate consequences. For example, consider the case of Frank, a runner who was preparing for the annual Mt. Marathon Race in Seward, Alaska. This

Fourth of July classic involves a 3,000' vertical ascent and descent on a peak with an average slope of 34 degrees. That's right, in places the course involves hand-over-hand climbing. Frank had done well the year before, finishing under an hour on his very first attempt. Given that his training had gone well, leaving him in much better shape than the year before, he seemed poised for a significant improvement.

Unfortunately, his mom came for a visit a few days before the event, purportedly to support him. (Think Klingon warships or the Trojan horse.) From the moment she arrived, Mom began criticizing Frank. This continued nearly non-stop for two days. Frank considered confronting mom about the attacks but concluded the most likely result would be a big fight and, based on past experience, he'd lose. Therefore, he chose to ignore the abuse and concentrate on his race instead.

That worked up until race time. As Frank described it a few days later: "From the start, I felt like I couldn't breathe. I never got my first wind, to say nothing of my second, like I usually do. My legs were heavy, like deadweight. I never really got going. People kept passing me. Last year, no one passed me once we hit the mountain. I was seven minutes slower than last year. What happened?"

As I worked on him, I discovered that Frank's respiratory diaphragm was drum-tight, probably from all that maternal criticism. This had interfered with the expansion and contraction of his lungs and heart, to say nothing about their visceral mobility and motility, virtually guaranteeing a sub-par performance. The contracted diaphragm would have interfered with his abdominal aorta and inferior vena cava and the arterial supply to his legs and venous and lymphatic return. His diaphragm also impeded liver and kidney motion and function, impairing energy supply and elimination of metabolic by-products such as lactic acid.

The messages implicit in mom's berating—"you're not good enough," "you're bad," "I don't love you," "you don't deserve to excel," "I'm jealous of you"—probably didn't help either. Indeed, a race is only a race. There is always next year, or not. However, the long-term impact of that content should be the real concern. In any event, given how much tension remained in Frank's diaphragm and abdomen, I thought he performed amazingly well on Mt. Marathon that year.

People tend to be quick to criticize athletes who fail to excel in big contests, disparaging them as "head-cases," "psyche-outs," "chokers," and the like. Unfortunately, given stress' effect on the respiratory diaphragm, "choking" is a relatively apt word choice. Combined with whatever else the athlete was dealing with, those situations may have overwhelmed the athlete's coping abilities, but the "choking" probably has as much or more to do with the stress reflex and somatomized content than any inherent character defect or weakness. The phrase that comes to mind here is: never criticize a person until you've walked (or run) a mile in his or her shoes.

Like Kudzu

Frank's story is all too common. I see evidence of the body-mind connection and the pernicious effects of somatomized content daily. For example, a patient complained of chronic pain and restrictions in her thoracic spine. On palpation, we felt an upward pull on her heart, as if it were stuck in her throat. She hadn't been in a relationship since her husband died a decade earlier. As she got in touch with her sorrow and loneliness, her chest became less rigid and her heart softened and became more motile.

Another patient was in so much pain that she could hardly move and walked as if she were frozen. As we treated her low back and shoulder pain, she disclosed that she'd put her life on hold a decade earlier to care for her husband after his heart attack. The husband had long since recovered and returned to motorcycling with his buddies, apparently without a backward look or word of appreciation. She had once been close to her daughter; however, now daughter only called when she needs "Grandma" to watch the grandkids. Obviously, the world had rewarded my patient's generosity with indifference, ingratitude, and a lack of reciprocity—a not atypical experience of those who are compulsive givers and caretakers.

This patient's frustration, disappointment, resentment, abandonment, and anger had landed in her body, causing multiple and painful restrictions. As she let go of those feelings, those restrictions melted. She began to move fluidly without pain and eventually resumed her bicycling for the first time in years. As she began re-making her life so that it worked for her, instead of for everybody else, husband and daughter became more considerate.

In addition to making and keeping us ill, somatomized content also contributes to accidents and injuries, as the following story suggests. A patient had never been injured or missed a day of work in more than 30 years. Then his grown son who'd always been so meticulous about firearm safety died while cleaning a handgun. Although the coroner declared the son's death an accident, dad couldn't be sure, as there were no witnesses. Understandably, the question became a major preoccupation, engendering guilt and self-doubt. A month after the son's death, dad injured himself on the job so badly and was in such pain that he'd had to have back surgery. The surgery had gone well and repaired the physical damage from the injury. But two months later, unrelenting pain left him unable to work. Was the timing of his injury a coincidence? We'll never know, but once he began talking about his son's death and released the associated feelings, his pain began to subside.

Somatomized content sets us up for injuries and illness two ways: it anchors us in dysfunctional pasts and acts as a major distraction. Content impairs our nervous system and decision-making. It may also activate genes that may lead to cancer and other diseases. One can imagine how continuously broadcast messages like: "I'm bad," I deserve to be punished," or "I'm in danger," There isn't enough of me to go around," or "I'm so angry!", can have serious negative consequences. These messages tend to be self-fulfilling. The previous examples should suffice, but more are scattered throughout subsequent chapters.

The US Center for Disease Control estimates that 85% of illness has an emotional component. Often, the emotional component was somatomized at some prior time. In other words, whether we know it or not, content in our tissues is probably messing with us. Innumerable examples illustrate the connection between body and mind. We'll get to more soon enough but, any way we look at it, we're dollars ahead—and a whole lot healthier— if we acknowledge that content may be involved and then roll up our sleeves to find and release it.

CHAPTER 9

How We Work with Content

Would You Like to Dance?

Given that patients are usually unaware that their tissues contain content, how do we find and release it? The simple answer is that much of the content lands in or creates mechanical restrictions—yet another reason why finding and releasing those restrictions is so important. When a restriction doesn't yield to gentle manipulation, content should always be suspected.

Restrictions leave the affected tissues feeling and looking different from surrounding tissues. The tissues might feel gummy, stagnant, or lifeless. The skin may appear dead white or drawn tight. We can ask the tissue if content is involved. If the patient is open to this technique, she will hear the tissue's answer.

Often, finding the restriction in a safe, therapeutic setting is all that is needed to release the associated content. Indeed, when the patient is ready to release content, we may have a hard time holding it back. For example, early in my career, before I'd learned that I could talk to the tissues, I was out on a house call. I'd been called by a friend because her tenant's back was in so much pain that she couldn't get up off the floor of her apartment. I knew she was a healthy, active young woman. She said she'd never had back problems previously. I spent an hour trying to release the spasms in her back muscles with every mechanical technique I knew.

Finally, in desperation, I asked her if she was on the anniversary of anything. After thinking for a minute, she said, "Oh, my God. A year ago, I was driving to Homer to give a talk. It was snowing. Visibility was poor. And we were stuck behind a truck. The truck slammed on its brakes and swerved. Too late. A woman had been walking in the roadway. The impact sent her flying, tore off her clothes, killed her instantly. There was nothing anybody could do. We were all in shock. Since we still had three more hours on icy roads ahead of us and others were willing to wait for the troopers with the truck driver, we left after about 15 minutes. But for more the next hour, I couldn't shake the image of that naked, battered body. I decided I had to focus on my talk. I guess I did a good job. I haven't thought about her lying in the snow for 12 months. It was horrible. What's today's date?"

"The 24th."

"Oh, my God, that was exactly a year ago, today. No wonder." Her back had started to relax the moment she started to telling me the story. By the time she finished, her pain was almost gone. I suggested she inhale some compassion for the dead woman, the trucker, herself, and everyone else there that day and exhale any cold, guilt, remorse, fear, anger, sadness, or other feelings that might have landed in her tissues. As she did, her remaining pain dissipated. She got up off the floor gingerly and asked me to run the tub for her before I left. When I saw her a few days later, she was fine.

Neither Rocket Science nor Brain Surgery

When patients are willing, my asking is the easiest way to learn if a restriction includes content. It's a simple question: "Is the restriction primarily physical, emotional, spiritual, or a combination?" If the answer is any of the last three options, we can ask a follow-up: "Would it be helpful (for the patient) to know any more about the restriction than we already do?" Often the answer to this last question is "no," meaning it's okay to just let the content go. If the answer is "yes," we keep asking more simple questions, such as: "How long has it been there? Show us something from back then that is related: a situation, event, person, or place? Is this content ours, another person's, or a combination?"

Sooner or later—and usually sooner, we arrive at the crossroads: is the patient willing to let go of the content? The answer is almost always "yes." If the answer is "maybe" or "no," we'll see if we can learn why and find a gentle way to "yes" by asking questions like "What it would take?" "What's the worst thing that could happen if you let go of this?" And so forth.

Usually, letting go of content boils down to patients giving themselves permission. Once they have, if they feel a need to do more, they can visualize letting it go, or they can exhale it from the tissue in question. If they believe that "nature abhors a vacuum," and they want to ensure that something undesirable doesn't move into the vacated space, they can replace the content with something positive, such as a sense of peace, acceptance, self-compassion, love, safety, courage, or strength. If this sounds simple, it is. Letting go of content is no more complicated than lifting the Mylar film on an Etch-a-Sketch when we're ready to change the doodle. The only difference is that the patient's mind and permission does the lifting.

Fear of Emotional Release Work

Some worry that exploring emotional content could unleash feelings and memories too strong to handle. It won't. Our egos—that part of our psyche focused on survival—won't permit that to happen. In fact, the greater likelihood is that our ego will prevent us from exploring and releasing content that we have been capable of handling for years. This is because the ego is all about being in control, and the more it's in control, the happier it is, even if its control is purchased with our health or even our life. This is the ultimate irony because one thing is for certain, when we die our ego dies too.

Fear is a normal, healthy reaction to potential danger. (Resistance, a common reaction to potential change, is slightly different and is explored at length in Chapter 12). Here is a summary of some the most common reasons that we fear emotional work: We were taught to fear emotions as children. We had primary caregivers who feared emotions and modeled burying their feelings. We were punished or shamed when we showed our feelings. We weren't safe. We knew adults who verbalized their feelings inappropriately, for example, by flying into a rage, harping, or complaining. Any one of these experiences might lead someone to conclude that feelings are bad or dangerous and should be suppressed, minimized, denied, or stuffed. Unfortunately, stuffing gives those same feelings even more power over us than they would have otherwise, and ignoring buried content is a recipe for illness.

Many cultures believe that showing or expressing feelings is a sign of weakness, especially in men. Of course, the opposite is true: working with content requires courage and strength, at least initially, but working with it soon makes us more resilient, more courageous, and stronger.

The over-dramatization of emotional release work in television and movies does not help. Emotional releases rarely involve drama or re-traumatization. This is true even when the original trauma was overpowering. Most emotional releases are routine, anticlimactic, and would be boring, if not for their significance to the patient's health.

For all these reasons and more, many people believe or would like to believe that their health challenge is entirely physical. While possible, this is rare. Indeed, the harder a person clings to this notion, the more likely it is that they are mistaken. Like anything new, working with content can be scary at first. But with a little practice, most people find releasing content is child's play.

Many people fear emotional release work, equating it with opening Pandora's box. It isn't. In fact, it's the opposite because that box was never closed. It has been broadcasting danger, negativity, or illness 24/7 to our brain and body since the moment of somatomization. Obviously, we can't change our history. But working with it in a therapeutic setting, we can deactivate the content, rendering it inert as far as the CNS is concerned so that it no longer keeps us stuck in fight-or-flight.

The Silver Lining

Using MRIs and PET scans, researchers at Harvard Medical School showed that when patients worked with somatomized content in a safe setting their amygdala and hippocampus became very active initially, putting the CNS in full alert. But after a few minutes when no actual danger materialized, the limbic system calmed down. And later, when patients revisited those memories, none of the physiological responses typically associated with fight-or-flight arose. In other words, working on content in a therapeutic setting deactivated it.

Other studies have found that stimulating acupuncture points in the presence of old trauma for a mere 15 minutes produced dramatic reductions in the levels of cortisol and other stress hormones in the subjects' blood. This also produced concurrent and equally dramatic reductions in phobias, anxiety, and PTSD.

In fact, with chronic, mysterious illness and pain, working with somatomized content may be the best hope for regaining health because it may be our body's attempt to get our attention. If, instead of tuning all this noise out or muffling it with medication or self-medication, we listen and take action, the body may no longer need to keep cranking up the volume with ever louder and more serious symptoms. Indeed, the pain may subside to manageable levels quickly.

Andrew Weil, MD, wrote over a dozen books on medicine, health, and natural healing. He was one of the first practitioners of and advocates for Integrative Medicine, which combines medicine with proven, evidence-based complementary and alternative approaches. The Integrative Medicine program at the University of Arizona Medical School, where Weil taught, is named after him. In *Spontaneous Healing*, one of his first books, published in 1995, he wrote that while medications may provide symptomatic relief temporarily, they often drive the problem deeper and produce more serious illnesses later.

There's almost always an elephant in the room—what's really up for us, some major issue that we're reluctant to talk about or lurking just below our conscious awareness. While many practitioners lack the time, inclination, or training to deal with this, the elephant is often the reason our symptoms and challenges aren't responding. Therefore, the sooner we acknowledge and deal with it the better because doing so can dramatically improve prognoses and speed recovery. Releasing content usually reduces our suffering.

I occasionally encounter people who believe that they've worked through all their issues. This is highly unlikely. In counseling or some other arena, they may indeed have worked through their more problematic stories, but not the associated content. Since somatomization is unconscious and automatic, it's nearly impossible to know what's in our tissues until we stumble upon it. This is one of the benefits of a systematic method for releasing restrictions in the tissues: it helps us find the content that often makes and keeps us ill and in pain.

Often when we find content in patients' tissues, they'll say something like, "Wow, I thought I'd worked through that." They may have worked through a related story in their mind. That's good, even helpful. It may mean that they're no longer fixated on it, and this usually makes releasing the content from the tissues that much easier. However, talk therapy alone is not likely to release the content from our tissues where it functions like the burr under the saddle. It needs to go.

Another argument for emotional work is that the lion's share of content probably originated with someone else. In other words, the content wasn't ours to begin with; we merely took it on, often from a family member, friend, person in authority, or coworker. Whether they projected it on to us, we took it on willingly, or some combination, we internalized it. This makes sense, as the word "overload" suggests that something has been put upon us. Indeed, Gary Douglas and Dr. Dain Heer, D.C., the founders of Access Consciousness®, a bodymind modality which has helped tens of thousands of people clear content out of their bodies, are fond of saying that 95% of somatomized content is actually not ours at all. The actual percentage hardly matters, but the possibility should motivate us to evict the content.

We take on other people's content for many reasons, ranging from altruism to naked self-interest, and often some combination.

We may want to help someone who is suffering. If we depend upon that person, we may believe that our welfare demands that we take on their stuff. Perhaps, our biology is the most important factor. Humans are social beings. Especially when we are young, our survival depends on our being accepted by the "tribe." Somatomization is one way we buy and maintain that acceptance. For example, if a child hears all day long that such and such a problem runs in the family, he is much more likely to internalize that belief and make it true for him too, rather than challenge the speaker and his belief and risk criticism, punishment, or rejection.

Innumerable stories illustrate the body-mind connection. For example, we traced one patient's neck and shoulder tension to the medulla oblongata (brain stem). The restriction felt old, pervasive. His head, neck and shoulders acted as if they were fused into a single inflexible structure. When I mentioned this, he explained that his x-rays showed degeneration in several vertebrae. While searching for the cause of his tension and pain, I employed the usual tricks: freeing up restrictions in the arteries and peripheral nerves of the neck. Traction. Acupressure. All helped a little but didn't release the restriction.

I followed the tension down his spine into his thoracic vertebrae. Unsure about exactly at which vertebral level we were working, I asked.

The moment he said, "Somewhere behind my heart," the tension let go; his shoulders relaxed, and his neck lengthened.

"What just happened?" I asked.

He said, "I just remembered. We had bunk beds growing up. One time my brother talked me into diving head first off the top bunk onto a pile of pillows. I didn't want to. I didn't trust him. But he kept trying. In the end, I dove. Then, while I was in mid-air, he jerked the pillows away."

"Lucky you didn't break your neck," I said.

"He was young, just a kid. He didn't know any better."

"Okay. Yes. But what emotions got stuck in your tissues?"

"I don't know," he said, then volunteered, "Surprise? Anger? Betrayal?"

"Whatever they are, would it be okay to let go of all of that today?" I asked, knowing he'd pretty much already just done that.

"It sure would," he said.

There was some softening in the thoracic vertebrae, but not enough. While I'm always obliged to make sure that we address the entire issue during a treatment, this is especially true where someone else has been intentionally injured because the patient may have consciously or otherwise taken on feelings that the injurer was trying to off load. "Did you take on any emotions from your brother at that time?" I asked.

"Oh? Wow! Yes, his anger. Some jealousy, too. But why would he...?"

"Would it be okay to let go of all of that now, too?" I asked.

"No problem!" he said.

"Would it be helpful to know any more about that than you are already consciously aware of today?"

"Nope!"

"Good, then please, go ahead and let it all go."

As he did, his back softened and neck relaxed. No wonder this person had degeneration in his cervical vertebrae! In addition to the physical force from the original injury, some of that damage may have stemmed from his conscious mind/ego trying to stuff emotions that, at one time, were too painful or unsafe to feel. Releasing all this gave his vertebrae a chance to heal and him a chance to avoid neck surgery.

This story also illustrates the ease and speed with which many patients uncover and release content. In that regard, it is typical. Much of the emotional content encountered during sessions is less memorable, but that makes it no less important in terms of our health. While some traumas strike us as worse than others, the nervous system has no relative scale for emotional trauma. For the bodymind, an event, comment, or interaction is either traumatic or it isn't.

Give Thanks for Somatomization

Whether a conscious choice or not, somatization is a brilliant survival strategy, as the following example suggests: "Becky" had almost died in a car accident. Open-heart surgery had saved her life. When I first saw her three years later, she was moving fairly well with the help of a cane. She was very positive, putting on a game face, but her pinched expression suggested she was in pain. We found a strong upward pull on her heart. After we released it and restored adequate blood supply to her brain, her face softened. By the end of the treatment, she looked radiant.

A year later, when I saw her next however, that pinched look was back. This time, we found a strong posterior-inferior tension pulling on her heart. It came from a restriction on the iliac vein in her left buttock. (The left and right iliacs return blood from the legs.) When I expressed some surprise and curiosity, she reminded me that her accident left her with two broken legs and that her surgeon had implanted mesh strainers in each vein to prevent blood clots from reaching her lungs. (This procedure has saved thousands of lives.) Once the danger had passed, the surgeon removed the sieves.

The restriction on the left responded to manual therapy and released in just a few minutes. When I rechecked however, there was still a strong inferior pull on Becky's heart, though now from her right buttock. Unlike the one on the left, however, the restriction on the right did not respond to purely manual efforts.

After several minutes, I asked her if the restriction was primarily physical, emotional, spiritual, or a combo?

Without hesitation, she said, "Spiritual: I'd been in the hospital for about a month. I was getting better, but ever so slowly, still in great pain, and quite weak. Lying there one day, it occurred to me that I might never again be the same as I had been prior to the accident."

"Would you be willing to let go of that attitude?" I asked.

As she was saying, "Sure! Why not?" the restriction released. Her gluteus muscles relaxed. On rechecking, the posterior inferior pull on her heart was gone. We restored her heart's motility, her face relaxed, her cheeks colored, and her whole body softened, just as it had the year before.

In one sense, part of Becky had spent an extra four years in that hospital bed, years that she'll never get back. It's unfortunate that patients who have been so physically traumatized rarely receive manual therapy. They usually get physical therapy, but too often that consists mostly of rehabilitation exercises. While beneficial, exercises are no substitute for releasing the associated energy, content and restrictions. Becky had not consciously somatomized those emotions. Indeed, as is usually the case, she wasn't even aware that she had, but it's easy to imagine how such a realization could constitute an overload.

As she lay in her hospital bed, however, the thought that she might be permanently damaged was simply too much for her to handle. At the very least, it would likely impede her recovery. Fortunately, her nervous system valet-parked the overload until she was ready for it, quite possibly sparing her from depression and a sense of defeat, which Becky could ill afford at that time when every ounce of her energy had been needed to fuel her recovery. Therefore, her brain somatomized the overload for a time when she would hopefully be better positioned to process it, or not. A brilliant and effective strategy.

Several years on, she had no resistance to letting go of this belief the moment she discovered it. Her willingness to jettison that old content was especially fortunate for her because, like the mind, mechanical restrictions, are rarely more deleterious than when they exert a significant drag on the heart. Ironically, owning and evicting the content moved her light-years closer to that once seemingly-impossible goal of regaining her former health, mobility, and vitality.

Osteopathic Approaches to Content:
Energy Cysts and SomatoEmotional Releases

While treating an energy cyst in a patient's liver, Dr. Upledger stumbled on the notion that the brain could park content in the tissues. His eyes were closed as he focused on feeling the tissues under his hands. The next thing he knew, the patient was pummeling him with her handbag.

His patient had suddenly gotten in touch with some old anger, couldn't distinguish it from her current circumstances, felt the need to express it, and found a convenient weapon in her purse and target in Dr. Upledger. Her anger had arisen spontaneously, not because of some agenda of Dr. Upledger. Indeed, this was an entirely new experience for him, one he'd never anticipated or sought. As if the universe wanted to be doubly sure that Dr. Upledger took note, a different patient released some buried emotions in a treatment a few days later. He later called these SomatoEmotional Releases (SERs).

Not surprisingly given his early experiences with SER, Upledger assumed that the bigger the drama—the more noise the patient made—the more significant the trauma and the associated release. However, he soon realized that the most significant releases were also usually the quietest and most subtle. A slight sigh, a tiny tear, or a slight softening of the area in question may be the only outward indication that a really important SER has occurred.

Some practitioners advertise that they do SERs, but this is inaccurate. Hopefully, they probably mean that they have some training and experience facilitating SERs. The patient does the SER. Therapists may find energy cysts and mechanical restrictions, but it's up to the patient to discover any associated content and let it go, or not.

Dr. Upledger wrote textbooks on SERs and collections of anecdotes from his clinical experiences. When first published in the 1980s, some of these stories seemed pretty astounding; they were for the time. In hindsight, however, to people familiar with SERs and the workings of the bodymind, most seem almost commonplace today.

Talking to the Tissues

Dr. Upledger was at his core a scientist. Indeed, he had done graduate studies in biochemistry prior to becoming an Osteopathic Physician. Therefore, he always insisted on understanding the science behind his discoveries. His book *Cell Talk: Stories Our Bodies Can Tell* marks a singular contribution to healthcare. In it, Dr. Upledger explains how DNA and RNA demonstrate a single cell's virtually unlimited information-storage capacity. From there, he discusses what he learned about the immune system and the substructures of the brain. Underlying all of these was Dr. Upledger's discovery, which we discussed in Chapter 6, namely that it is possible—and extremely productive—to talk directly to the tissues.

A Light Bulb Goes on

Until very recently when new imaging techniques became available, much of what science knew about the brain's substructures stemmed from what functions were affected or lost following strokes, injuries, and tumors. Focused on mundane but critical matters like life, death, cognition, language, and memory, most neurologists understandably ignored more esoteric but nonetheless significant functions, many of which have to do with our peace of mind.

Wondering if the substructures of the CNS might possibly perform services that medicine was unaware of, Upledger began to ask these structures what they did and what their purpose was. In reply, the structures soon revealed functions that other physicians had never contemplated. Sensing he may have stumbled upon a therapeutic gold mine and wanting to be sure he wasn't making things up or missing anything important, Upledger taught colleagues and students these techniques and encouraged them to keep records of what they learned.

The resultant data confirmed his findings and filled in many blanks. For example, science knew that the corpus callosum fosters communication between right and left hemispheres. The researchers discovered that the corpus callosum also balances logic and emotion. Based on what we know about right brain/left brain, that wasn't too surprising. However, Upledger may have been the first to use this information to help patients who had previously been excessively emotional or logical.

The fornix is a slingshot-shaped midbrain structure folded nearly into a circle. Science knew that the fornix serves an important role in memory. Under questioning, numerous fornixes revealed that they were also responsible for trust. Working with the fornix has helped patients regain their ability to trust.

The pituitary gland and the glabella (an area of the frontal bone between the eyebrows) reported that they function as the brain's pharmacies. Once their needs are met, the glabella and pituitary theoretically can regulate the production of any chemical the CNS needs. The pineal glands, which help control circadian rhythms, told Upledger that they obtain their energy through a bone in the roof of the mouth (vomer) and the temples (sphenoid), giving us another tool in the treatment of sleep disturbances like insomnia and jet lag.

Furthermore, Upledger learned that adults who hadn't cut the apron strings often had mom "stuck" in their pituitary. Whether this is a metaphor, mom's energy, or some unmet need for maternal love is academic. What matters is that the situation impairs pituitary function, possibly disrupting the entire endocrine system. Not surprisingly, it also complicates the mother-child relationship for both parties. Typically, after a "mom" has been evicted, the relationship improves almost instantaneously. As if that weren't sweet enough, improving the pituitary's space and addressing its other needs may also resolve a host of endocrine challenges. Good, bad, or indifferent, the maternal relationship is critical to a person's development, subsequent launch, and trajectory.

Again, the benefits of this single pituitary discovery cut two ways. Mother issues may be a clue that the pituitary is challenged. Conversely, an endocrine challenge may indicate unresolved maternal issues. In either case, manual therapy can help resolve those issues and diminish their health consequences.

It Takes a Village

Some CNS structures seem to have distinct personalities and voices. As mentioned before, the hypothalamus is extremely busy and therefore may sound curt or gruff. If I ask a patient's hypothalamus if it will speak with us, I'm likely to hear something like "Whaddaya want?" Another structure might respond with something less irritated like "Sure, I thought you'd never ask!" or "It's about time!" The tone can vary from humorous to frustrated, even nearly defeated, depending on the patient's and the structure's situation.

Initially, patients may not be able to tell whether the structure answering is the one they are trying to work with or the cerebral cortex. That's okay. Answers that begin with "I think" suggest that the cerebral cortex or ego is talking, not the structure we addressed. We probably don't want to listen to the ego, however; if the cortex turns out to be the talker, we shouldn't automatically dismiss what it says. There's nothing fundamentally wrong with the cortex. Indeed, it brims with intelligence. In the long run, what matters is not which structure gets the credit, but that the job gets done.

In God, We Trust (All Others Pay Cash!)

While the previously mentioned structures are familiar to anatomists and neurologists, this is not the case with centrum, which may be more of a function than a distinct physical structure, akin to acupuncture meridians whose existence and locations are accepted, even though no meridian has ever been dissected. I doubt that anyone has used a functional MRI to document centrum at work, as has been done with most other structures. However, centrum has told us where it is and what it does, so we can guess approximately which tissues it inhabits.

Think of centrum as an internal antenna from the center of the forehead to the base of the skull and down the spinal cord to the level of the heart. Centrum has told us that it functions as our direct, personal up-link with the divine. As such, centrum can be a source of almost impeccable personal advice because it knows our personal spiritual path. It can be especially helpful when we are confused, stuck, wrestling with a dilemma, or distrust our intuition. I turn to it often, especially if I can't resist suggesting a course of action.

Centrum's guidance is not generic, but personally tailored to us. This guidance differs from advice from friends, family members, priests, counselors, physicians, or manual therapists. While often full of common sense and well intentioned, their advice might be wrong for us. In contrast, centrum's suggestions usually resonate with us, making them all the more likely to be followed. Most patients who have talked to centrum seem to accept that it exists and have found its advice extremely helpful.

Gaining access to centrum—both as a resource and source of independence—can dramatically accelerate a person's journey from illness to health and from victim to survivor. The discovery that we have a reliable internal guidance system can be extremely reassuring and empowering, especially when we are used to ignoring or distrusting our own intuition. During treatments, centrum can also keep us from wasting time exploring rabbit trails.

The Bottom Line

CNS structures have four basic needs: adequate space, blood, cerebrospinal fluid, and energy. While these requirements may seem self-evident, medicine generally does not focus on them, except in acute situations and, more importantly, has few ways of addressing them. On the other hand, in non-emergency situations, manual therapists can usually address these shortcomings.

Visceral Manipulation and the BodyMind

Dr. Barral developed some extremely simple yet sophisticated techniques for treating the bodymind. These include discovering emotional circuit breakers in the gastrointestinal tract and developing techniques for diagnosing and treating their malfunctions. He also developed manual techniques for detecting and treating energetic, emotional, and spiritual disturbances.

Dr. Barral and his collaborators have also made some of the most significant new contributions to the understanding of the relationships between specific internal organs and the emotions since the advent of Traditional Chinese Medicine. Based on more than 60,000 of Dr. Barral's treatments, these are summarized in *Understanding the Messages of Your Body: How to Interpret Physical and Emotional Signals to Achieve Optimal Health*.

As the description of Visceral Manipulation techniques in the previous chapter suggests, Dr. Barral's and his colleagues' abilities to feel what is going on in body tissues is phenomenal. This manual acuity stems from an encyclopedic familiarity with anatomy combined with God-given gifts developed over decades of practice. Despite being able to spot restrictions on individual organs from across the room, Dr. Barral always confirms what he's seen with his hands. His willingness to trust his senses makes it possible for his skills to blossom even further. As a result, he occasionally finds incipient tumors and malignancies that MRIs and CT-scans have missed.

Emotional Circuit Breakers

Early in his development of Visceral Manipulation, Dr. Barral noticed that some of the one-way valves in the gastrointestinal tract occasionally went into spasm. Eventually, he concluded that five of those one-way valves were prone to spasm when a person experienced an emotional overload. Most people won't notice one of these emotional circuit breakers pop. However, by the next day, they will often experience acute abdominal pain, throbbing headaches, or flu-like symptoms. Difficult to ignore, the discomfort can engender considerable worry. Some patients try to tough it out. Some self-medicate. Others seek medical attention. None of these strategies is very effective, although ruling out something serious can be reassuring.

It is possible to manually detect the spasms and reset the valves, thus avoiding thousands of dollars in emergency room visits and tests and hours of pain and worry. Furthermore, in the process of treating the spasm, the person may realize what caused the overload in the first place and release the associated content. When in spasm, the overlying tissues rotate counterclockwise immediately upon palpation. When not in spasm, the overlying tissue will be stationary or rotate clockwise initially. Armed with this information, Dr. Barral developed several techniques for releasing the spasms and re-setting the valves.

Assuming they show no signs of having a medical emergency such as appendicitis, when patients present with these sudden-onset symptoms, we listen to the tissues overlying the sphincters. While manually treating a spasm in one of these valves, I'll usually ask the patient if something upsetting happened the day before. Frequently, patients will then remember having had their buttons pushed. The trigger could be as simple as seeing a cat or dog darting across a busy street in the face of oncoming traffic, seeing an adult roughly treat an obstreperous child at the supermarket, witnessing an argument or altercation, or having our spouse ignore our advice and then later complain bitterly when the outcome we predicted materialized.

For example, a naturopath sent me a patient with dangerously high blood-sugar levels, telling me that I was the last hope short of insulin medication with all its undesirable side effects. On palpating his abdomen, my hand was attracted to his sphincter of Oddi, a valve at the duodenal end of the end of the bile duct. When functioning properly this valve prevents bile and digestive enzymes from the gall bladder and pancreas from reaching the small intestine when they are not needed. Oddi was in spasm and leaking, due to tension coming from his pancreas. Apparently contact with his mother had rekindled some frustration from childhood. After he released the content from his pancreas and we reset his sphincter of Oddi, his blood sugar levels normalized.

When one of these valves is in spasm, manual therapy usually resets the sphincter and dissipates the symptoms within minutes. From a practitioner's point of view, being able to relieve acute problems so quickly is extremely rewarding. When it comes to convincing people of the validity and utility of the body-mind connection, successfully resetting a sphincter is tough to match. As an added bonus, patients can learn how to recognize and self-treat these spasms.

While temporarily debilitating, the short-term consequences of the spasm may be the least of the problem. For example, Chapter 3 discussed how a spasm in the valve between the esophagus and the stomach could lead to Gastro-Esophageal Reflux Disorder (GERD). In addition to producing pain, GERD can murder sleep, burn the esophagus, and lead to esophageal cancer. At the other end of the GI tract, another valve, the ileocecal, prevents fecal matter from the cecum, the first part of the colon, from backflowing into the ilium, the small intestine. Spasms in the ileocecal valve may lead to appendicitis, which is life threatening.

A few years before I learned about these emotional circuit breakers and their spasms, I experienced acute pain in my lower right abdomen. I had been working on some of my childhood issues at the time and was prepared to ride out the pain in hopes it would diminish. However, my partner, who was out of town had different ideas. Years before, her brother, not realizing he was suffering from acute appendicitis, had ignored his abdominal pain and nearly died from infection after his appendix ruptured. Fearing I might be next, and unable to see with her own eyes that I wasn't seriously ill, she threatened to call 911 if I didn't go to the hospital immediately. Therefore, I went.

The resident on duty in the ER couldn't find anything wrong: x-rays were negative, vital signs were normal, and my abdomen wasn't unusually rigid or tender on palpation. But from a medical perspective, these results only added to the mystery. Over the next few hours, the resident palpated my abdomen several times. Each time he did, the pain subsided a little bit more. However, wanting to be absolutely sure he hadn't missed something critical before releasing me, he had me wait for the internist on-call who was performing a surgery.

After about four hours, the surgeon finally arrived. Apologizing for the wait, he mumbled something about complications. Indeed, he looked like he'd been through the wringer. After asking questions and palpating my abdomen, he announced that everything seemed normal. At which point, trying to be helpful, I suggested that my malaise might have had something to do with the childhood trauma I was working through. His response was simple: "I've opened up thousands of abdomens over the years and have never found an emotion in one yet." Then he sent me home. Twenty-five years later, I still have my appendix.

The resident had probably never heard about the connection between emotions and sphincters at the time. Two years passed before I learned about it in a workshop. However, in retrospect, I'm convinced that his palpations released a spasm in my ileocecal valve. Who knows, he may have even spared me appendicitis and an appendectomy. I'd known a chiropractor who claimed he could head off appendicitis by using his activator (those spring-loaded T-shaped stainless-steel devices that chiropractors use to deliver force to specific vertebrae) on the ileocecal valve. Crude, compared to Dr. Barral's methods but, sometimes we get lucky.

Lord of the Ring

Chapter 6 mentioned the energy fields surrounding our physical body. Not surprisingly, Visceral Manipulation has techniques for finding and treating leaks in these energetic shells resulting from somatomized content. When I was in a workshop learning about these techniques, my practice mate found a thermal projection in the emotional envelope near my stomach. She moved the energy up into my head and silently asked my body to show her a picture of the problem. Shortly thereafter, she asked if a ring held any meaning for me. As nothing sprang to mind, I asked her to describe it. She said it looked like an engagement ring and featured a large sapphire surrounded by two pearls set in a ring of tiny diamonds.

I was stunned. My mother's! Without further prompting, I immediately remembered something I'd completely forgotten: about 40 years earlier, I'd picked up the ring off of my mother's desk and absent-mindedly pocketed it my Little League trousers. An hour later standing in in centerfield, I was shocked to find the ring in my pocket. A welter of fear and panic arose. My parents' marriage had always felt pretty rocky to me and, based on their arguments, I assumed I was a significant cause, as kids often will. Now, I worried their marriage might not survive the loss of that ring. I had no safer place to keep it. I was never much good at baseball, that day especially, and was never gladder than when that game ended. Somehow, I managed to return the ring to my mom's dresser without being discovered. As we often do, I'd apparently buried the memory and associated panic and fear. My parents' marriage survived another decade until cancer took my father.

I was impressed. In 40 years, I had never thought about that situation again nor mentioned it to anyone. Ever. I released the associated feelings, and the therapist moved the energy, which was no longer chaotic, out of my head and into nerve junctions in my abdomen. Even though I hadn't been aware of having carried a burden, I could feel my whole body relax. Among other things, the exercise was a great example of how we unconsciously dump emotional overloads into our tissues so that we are able to keep functioning—and how seemingly mundane the vast majority of this content can be when we re-encounter it years later.

Working with the bodymind to clear afflictive emotions from the tissue pays big dividends. However, our next topic, using manual therapy to find and address spiritual injuries, may be even more important.

CHAPTER 10

Spirit: Coming Home

One of manual therapy's most important applications is healing the human spirit. In this context, spirit has nothing to do with religion and everything to do with our relationship with ourselves. While personal growth and spiritual healing may at first strike many readers as a luxury or self-indulgence for the affluent only, it's a necessity for most everyone. Many who can least afford it need it most. Would you rather be with people who feel good about themselves or with people who don't?

Arguably, nothing affects our health more than a spiritual wound. When we feel bad about ourselves, we're more likely to get sick and injured, engage in self-defeating behaviors, and do things we later regret. Self-judgment also impedes recovering from illness, injuries, and surgeries. Indeed, spiritual injuries and issues are the root of many chronic health challenges. Therefore, the sooner we find and release spiritual content, the better and the more likely we are to attain deep, lasting health.

Emotional wounds equate with hurt feelings. These are bad enough. Spiritual wounds result in our feeling fundamentally flawed. This belief is far more destructive than emotional wounds as it suggests that we deserve to be punished. If that's what we think, we will experience punishment of one or more forms: health, financial, legal, relational, and so forth.

For example, one patient had several chronic health challenges and a ton of pain. A decade prior, he had committed a serious crime while on medication. His psychotherapist had misdiagnosed him and prescribed the wrong medication. The patient could tell the medication was wrong, but his psychotherapist wouldn't listen and insisted that he keep taking his medicine. Therefore, he had not been in his right mind at the time of his crime, but after his arrest, he felt so ashamed of and guilty about what he'd done that he refused to mount a defense or enlighten his public defender. Therefore, the psychotherapist never testified. Ignorant of the mitigating circumstances, the court handed down a sentence of seven years.

The patient had been out of prison three years when we started working together intermittently. His symptoms usually improved after each treatment but never completely disappeared. After several weeks or a month, his pain would return, usually with a vengeance. After four years of working together occasionally, I assumed that his self-judgment had gradually softened and suggested to him that he had suffered enough.

Judging from his reaction, I was wrong. End of conversation. Apparently the seven years of hard time and seven more years of self-imposed incarceration weren't enough in his mind. The walls went up. End of therapeutic relationship. Nothing I could say made the slightest difference. He essentially fired me on the spot.

I'd finally found the elephant in the room, and I had to respect it, even though it meant that there was little more that I or anyone else could do for this patient, until and unless his attitude changed. By various means, he made it clear that that wasn't likely. Obviously, my patient believed that his crime was unforgivable and therefore he was intent on serving a lifetime of self-imprisonment.

What's Love Got to Do with It

Louise L. Hay, author of the self-help classic *You Can Heal Your Life*, believed that all illness stems from a lack of self-acceptance and self-love. Years ago, when I first read this, I thought Dr. Hay's theory was a little simplistic, perhaps true for some, but not for everyone. Three decades of clinical experience later, however, I believe she was more right than wrong. Time and again, when patients don't get well, self-judgment is often in play. That was almost always the case with my military patients.

Even the most fortunate among us have experienced traumas that have damaged our relationship with ourselves. While we may not remember the trauma or recognize it for what it is, our tissues do, and they keep reminding our Central Nervous System (CNS) about it. Manual therapy can help us find and evict that content so that we can heal our spirit and regain our health.

Restrictions and Symptoms as Buried Treasure

Typically, medicine tries to eradicate illness and symptoms as quickly as possible, as if they had no inherent value. This is understandable: That is what doctors are expected to do. We all want to be well yesterday, and nobody more so than someone who is really ill or badly injured. However, illness and pain may be wake-up calls, signals that a gap exists between where we are on our spiritual path and where we should be. We often miss this message because we've been taught to medicate and eliminate, suppress symptoms or undergo surgery on the offending part. When we do, we may miss an opportunity to heal something of great importance, something that may otherwise come back later with a vengeance. That alone should persuade us to engage more fully with our symptoms.

Louise Hay saw the metaphysical implications of various symptoms: for example, a bad knee might indicate a challenge with moving forward; chronic shoulder pain might result from a belief that we are carrying the weight of the world; and so forth. For each, she prescribed a specific, curative new belief to use as a mantra or affirmation. For example, for the shoulder, it would be, "I choose to allow all my experiences to be joyous and loving."

Ms. Hay may have been one of the earliest, but she was far from alone in believing that a lack of self-love and self-acceptance underlay all illness. The late Ron Kurtz, PhD, co-founder of Hakomi Body-Centered Psychotherapy, did too. Kurtz's methodology was quite simple: Listen to the patient's story for a few minutes, distill it down to its essence, and form the most specific nutritive statement possible. This would be some variant of "You're lovable just the way you are." After the patient turned inwards, Kurtz would feed him this prompt while observing closely. Typically, some almost imperceptible and non-conscious body response would be the clue that that the patient felt otherwise and wouldn't allow himself to believe that this might be true. If the patient was not aware of this response, Kurtz would have him turn inward again and repeat the process. Bringing this gesture or mannerism to the patient's attention would raise the underlying issue to consciousness where it could then be resolved.

Absent a great deal of inner work, most of us are playing a similar tape in our mind 24/7. If we are, we might as well replace it with something affirming our innate worthiness. This is especially true if, at first, that is *not* how we feel and what we believe about ourselves. Those negative beliefs—that we are fundamentally flawed—are most likely hard-wired, and it will take some effort to replace them with healthier ones. Therefore, the sooner we start, the better. Many of us will balk at the apparent self-indulgence of repeating a mantra that affirms our inherent self-worthiness. The more we resist, however, the more we're likely to need it.

Similarly, the famous psychiatrist Sir David Hawkins, MD, viewed mental illness as a symptom of a great spiritual injury. Often, he was able to eradicate extremely intractable conditions simply by a prolonged, non-judgmental gaze directly into the patient's eyes. Very few people have worked on themselves enough to be able to gaze non-judgmentally into another person's eyes. I'm guessing that this is especially true with patients suffering from serious mental illness because few maladies are so unsettling and triggering. Hawkins was neither the first to be able to do this nor will he be the last. Nonetheless, the fact that he did can inspire us to roll up our sleeves and work on our issues. The restrictions in our tissues can guide us to the material we need for our upgrade.

Another leading psychotherapist, Arthur Mindell, PhD, also viewed symptoms as indications of a gap between our spiritual blueprint and our spiritual attainment. In his book *Working with The Dreaming Body*, Mindell wrote, "Your scariest symptoms may be your greatest dream trying to come true."

Mindell was not advocating foregoing medical care. Instead, he was suggesting that we should engage with our illness to see if it's trying to tell us something. In my experience, if there is a message and we discover it, the symptoms or illness are likely to abate and not return. Since many symptoms arise from mechanical restrictions, many of which include somatomized content, we can imagine how finding and releasing restrictions might be part of a spiritual path. When we have a challenge, a particularly germane question might be, "What's right about this that I'm not getting?"

Many philosophers believe that our primary purpose on the planet is healing spiritual wounds. If so, one can see the potential benefit of working with symptoms, at least until we fully understand them. To learn if the symptom, illness, or restriction has a message, I will ask, when patients are willing. The process and techniques are identical to those discussed for emotional content in the previous chapter. Only the results differ: the healing is not just on physical and emotional levels, but on our relationship with ourself.

Understandably, for patient and practitioner alike, the first inclination will always be to rid the body of symptoms and disease. However, the symptom or disease may have information critical to the patient's long-term health, welfare, survival, and life's purpose. If we can momentarily resist the elimination urge and instead engage the symptoms or tissues in conversation, we may learn something vitally important. If we do and the patient acts on this new insight, healing usually follows.

Many of us were damaged in shipping and handling (childhood), some of us severely. As a result, we often draw the wrong conclusions about ourselves and proceed accordingly. That merely compounds our suffering and fosters addictions and other ills. These maladaptions tend to persist unless and until the associated pain becomes so unbearable that we say "Uncle!" and seek help.

Ain't No Sunshine When You're Gone

There's a certain consolation in being a victim, even if it's hollow. With victims, nothing is ever their fault, and they never have to take responsibility for their choices. (To be clear, I'm not blaming victims. There are many situations where people had no choice. It's not a perfect world. Bad things happen.) However, over time, victims tend to burnish the original spiritual injury and attract more. In this sense, a single spiritual wound can morph into great spiritual self-violence.

Early in this chapter, I wrote about a patient who committed a serious crime. Do you think he had a perfect childhood? Probably not. Indeed, his was pretty horrific. In such cases, children often assume that bad things happened to them because they were bad and deserved it. Abusers often plant such notions and cultivate them as a way of avoiding their own guilt and culpability and keeping victims groomed and primed for more victimization. (Unfortunately, it's a fairly effective and extremely common strategy.) A victim may be old enough to be a grandparent yet, for all intents and purposes, still stuck in an abusive childhood. Hence, no sunshine.

Self-judgment is completely antithetical to self-love. It's impossible to love yourself and judge yourself simultaneously. Yet many of us are world champion self-judgers. Self-judgment almost invariably leads to self-loathing and self-punishment. This is why I've concluded that Louise Hay was correct, that most illness stems from a lack of self-love and self-acceptance. If so, one can see the wisdom of self-compassion: it can unlock the cell of self-punishment and spring us from self-imprisonment.

Painful and debilitating as they may be, physical, emotional, and spiritual challenges may also be our greatest treasures when they compel us to look within. Because our history is in our tissues, bodywork is one of the most promising paths and expressways to spiritual healing. With each piece of somatomized content that we release, we move further from victimhood, while gaining strength, skills, courage, clarity, and health. Moreover, the mere act of rolling up our sleeves to work on content implicitly acknowledges and honors our own self-worthiness. That alone can be a significant step toward health. Each piece of emotional, spiritual, and psychic content that we release brings us closer to our essence, our innate perfection, which is divine.

It Ain't Over, 'til It's Over

"If we can fog a mirror," goes the expression, "There is still hope." Manual therapy's promise stems from its ability to find and free up mechanical restrictions, including those with content. Because manual therapists typically spend more time with each patient than most doctors can, and everything (physical, emotional, and spiritual) is on the table, the manual therapist often has a much better chance of finding and resolving the root of the problem, instead of just managing or medicating it. Best of all, the pot of gold at the end of the journey is none other than us.

In *Daring Greatly*, Brené Brown, PhD, compares the toxic, paralyzing nature of shame to the rewards of vulnerability. She argues that it is better to try (which entails vulnerability) and to fail, than not to try at all. Ironically, in her professional career, Professor Brown did everything she could to avoid the spotlight and the associated vulnerability. It found her anyway, as so often happens. There must be a law of nature that says that the harder we try to avoid something, the more likely it's going to occur. The story of Oedipus is one of the first written on the topic.

In her earlier book *The Gifts of Imperfection*, Brown describes the character traits common to highly successful people. She notes that these people accept their imperfections, refrain from self-judgment, practice self-compassion, learn from their mistakes, and move on. In other words, we don't need to be alchemists to turn our trauma into gold; it already is, and we are, too. For most of us, it will take some effort to get to where we can see that. For those of us not sufficiently adept or practiced to do all of that personal work on our own, it's okay to ask for help.

Sitting on Dynamite

The following example shows that working with spiritual content is no different from working with emotional content: Working with a patient one day, I noticed that each inhalation was jamming his head down on his cervical vertebrae (a classic sign of a lung restriction, discussed in Chapter 4.) We tracked the problem down to the respiratory diaphragm's attachments to his lumbar spine. As we freed up the fascia in the area, I asked his body how long the associated restriction had been there.

The answer was "All my life."

I asked, "Body, is this tension mostly physical, emotional, or spiritual?"

"Spiritual," he said.

"Ask your body to show you what this is about."

"My dad. The way he treated me. He was horrible. As an infant, I just assumed that I wasn't worthy of love: That I was unlovable. I guess part of me must still feel that way. Wow! That certainly explains a lot."

"Would it be okay to let go of that today?"

"Sure."

My patient had been living with this pattern for more than 60 years. As a grown man, he'd come to understand what he hadn't realized as a small child, namely that his dad's behavior had little to do with him and everything to do with his dad. That insight had been helpful but hadn't released the belief that he was unlovable from where it was parked in his tissue. Therefore, his head continued to pound down on his cervical vertebrae with each inhalation. As I helped my patient let go of this belief, his lower back and diaphragm softened, his breathing eased, the pounding of his head on his cervical spine decreased, and he moved closer to reclaiming his inherent self-worth and divinity.

Spiritual content can be devastating. When we believe that we are unlovable or unworthy of love, despite our best intentions, we infallibly find people who will treat us shabbily and reinforce that belief. Such beliefs are exceedingly wearing and account for many illnesses, accidents, depressions, and suicides.

Health and Healing as a Spiritual Path

When we begin to mend our relationship with ourselves, we tend to stay healthy and avoid injuries. When we understand and work through our spiritual injuries, illnesses may "evaporate like dew in the morning sun."

Somatomized content is almost always at play when we experience chronic problems. Indeed, there may be many layers of it. Therefore, if the symptom doesn't relent or the illness doesn't abate, don't give up. Keep going. Each layer that is released brings us closer to our goal. Health is as much a journey as a destination. Our culture is so organized around instant gratification that we often forget that many things, healing among them, take time. I, too, would like to see every patient get better yesterday. This does happen occasionally, but usually not. When healing appears to be spontaneous, the patient has probably been laying the groundwork for a considerable period of time beforehand.

Over several years, "Heidi" went from being chronically ill with a port in her chest to facilitate the injection of medicine directly into her venous system to being mostly healthy and medication free. Depending on the season, she is now able to hike, ski, and snowshoe.

Of course, having been so sick for so long, she is not yet as strong as she's going to be. In some ways, this history makes her the proverbial canary in the coalmine, where she's more sensitive to stress and pollution than the average person. For example, moving out of her condo into a new home took its toll. This is not surprising because moving can be stressful for even the strongest and healthiest person. All that packing, cleaning, lifting, and disruption of normal routines and diet exacted even more of a toll on Heidi than it would on most people. That in turn, left her more vulnerable to the inevitable construction dust and out-gassing of new building materials in her new home.

Heidi's primary complaint of the day was apparent when she walked into my office just after finishing her move: she was unable to turn her head or hold it upright. Her neck was frozen at about 10 degrees forward. We started by freeing up her new lung restrictions—from the dust and cleaning products. Then we unjammed her occiput so it could return to its normal place atop her first cervical vertebrae. Her brain was a quart low on arterial blood and Cerebrospinal Fluid (CSF). Once we restored adequate arterial blood and CSF supply and circulation to her brain, she felt 75% better than when she'd walked in, and she could turn her head more than 60 degrees in both directions.

Heidi returned a few days later, feeling much better, but her head and neck were still forward and her throat tight. There was considerable tension in her stomach; its lesser curve was very tight. This is quite common with patients who've experienced a great deal of criticism or indulged in significant amounts of self-criticism because the solar plexus area seems to be a favorite repository for both.

When it comes to talking to her body, Heidi is a rock star. When restrictions don't respond to manual therapy, she usually finds and addresses the associated content very quickly. This time was no exception. She was able to track the problem down to the stress of moving and having drunk a can of soda, against her better judgment. Once she'd found and let go of the stress and associated issues, her stomach began to relax. Stretching her esophagus relieved the tension in her throat and allowed her head to relax backward into a more normal position.

Even so, the muscles connecting her left occiput to her left shoulder remained unacceptably tight. After her body informed us that this was related to her cycle, we traced this problem to a hormone shortage stemming from the thalamus crowding the hypothalamus. She released the associated issues and the muscles relaxed. This did not eliminate all of Heidi's long-standing endocrine challenges, but it was an important step in that direction.

Thyroid challenges are notoriously difficult to resolve using medications. For starters, getting the dosage exactly correct is often critical. I know smart people who have resorted to razor blades to slice the pills into the right number of milligrams. Too much or too little and they experience huge mood swings. And then of course, the throat is a rough neighborhood. Like the thymus gland several inches below, the thyroid's needs are always going to be sacrificed to address the brain's and heart's needs for blood and space.

Cat Got Your Tongue?

Speaking of the thyroid, the throat is so important for self-expression that Dr. Upledger named it "the avenue of expression." Unfortunately, from an early age, many of us were discouraged from speaking our mind and encouraged to stuff our needs and feelings. Typically, this results in a great deal of mechanical tension in the throat and around our thyroid. Once established, this self-censorship often persists, unless and until the person becomes aware of it and is driven to change it. When self-censorship has been a survival strategy, this may take decades. By then, a whole chain of endocrine imbalances may be in play. Since the medical consequences are so serious, the tendency to treat the symptoms without giving a moment's thought to their cause is understandable.

There's no quicker way to damage a child's spirit than telling her repeatedly that everything about her is wrong. That had been the message Heidi received every day while growing up. She was a tomboy with a stepdad who believed that girls should be sugar and spice and all things nice, wear girlie clothes, and act like Prissy Missy. With no support from her mom, she had been in no position to confront her stepdad and therefore ended up with considerable tension around her thyroid. Like their owners, thyroids don't thrive under gag orders and the associated buried emotions and mechanical tensions.

When we have a challenge, we should always look for the cause. In addition to self-censorship, many thyroid problems, stem from mechanical imbalances on adjacent structures such as arteries, nerves, lungs, or even the esophagus or challenges further upstream in the endocrine system (the hypothalamus and pituitary). Thyroid issues could also stem from being stuck in fight-or-flight. Resolving those issues might obviate much of the need for thyroidectomies and hormonal supplementation.

There were at least three reasons why Heidi had fallen prey to her environmental exposures during her move. First, there was the stress of moving itself. Secondly, she had had no time for her normal stress management practices, especially her above-tree line, spirit-buoying hikes with her dogs. This alone was a double-whammy because the bad indoor air quality had been exacerbated by a prolonged thermal inversion which had blanketed Anchorage with road dust, pollen, and vehicular emissions. Hiking above that inversion layer would have had her breathing hard, exhausting the toxins, replacing them with fresh, relatively pristine air, and given her a couple hours' break from inhaling that toxic soup.

In the course of 30 treatments over two years with me, Heidi probably released a hundred restrictions that had been held in place by content. Many had not been hers to begin with but belonged to her parents. She'd previously worked through many of these issues during counseling. However, that had mainly focused on the narrative in her head while the content, the history, had remained in her tissues. Despite the indignities that she'd suffered and their debilitating consequences, nothing ever arose during her treatments during all that time that we worked together that she couldn't handle.

Parked emotions and beliefs are essentially only energy. Releasing that energy rarely involves reliving the original trauma. Indeed, most of the time we don't even need to know what the content is or what it's about; we merely need to give ourselves permission to let go of it. This was generally true for Heidi. Usually, her answer to the question "Would it be helpful to know any more about this than we are already consciously aware of?" was "No." This reaffirms my point that healing is mostly about permission, less about remembering or understanding and almost never about re-experiencing.

Theoretically, all of us should be able to find and release our content on our own. Indeed, I believe this often occurs during meditation. But for a host of reasons—personal, familial, and cultural—this is not always possible, especially when we are ill or have been so for a long time. When illness has become our default mode, it is nice to have a little extra help. Often, all we need is someone who knows what questions to ask and what order to ask them in. When we're sick, a manual therapist can provide the extra energy and safety we need to find the elephants in the room, identify them for what they are, and send them packing.

Finding and evicting those elephants is so important because buried content anchors us in a problematic past; keeps us in some degree of fight-or-flight; and maintains mechanical restrictions and the associated pathology. This is especially true in the case of spiritual injuries. According to the law of inertia, bodies resist changes in their status: a body in motion tends to stay in motion, and so forth. We can expect that a body in illness will tend to remain in illness, absent some sort of input. That is why we often need a little help. Many hands make light work. In that sense, the therapist can help arrest the patient's downward spiral, propel a patient in stasis toward healing, and accelerate the movement toward health.

For more than two decades of constant parental criticism, Heidi has paid a very high price, and her health is not yet perfect, but it improves. Moreover, thanks to her courage and her self-acceptance, she is able to find the content and release it. She's one of my heroines.

"Venus" is another. She had had a horrific childhood, filled with every kind of abuse. Not surprisingly, she then experienced several, far-from-perfect marriages. Although she'd worked through a lot of that, she'd been brutally assaulted shortly before we met. You'd never guess this from looking at or speaking to her, thanks to the miracles of modern medicine, a wonderful surgeon, an indomitable spirit, and lots and lots of personal work.

Long before we met, Venus had been focusing on bringing ever more compassion and love for herself and others. Therefore, she was content when we started and has grown increasingly so. In my presence, she's released hundreds of restrictions. Since I'm not her only manual therapist, I can only assume she's probably let go of several times that number with her other practitioners. More than half of the restrictions we released were in her lungs. Although she wasn't even aware of them beforehand, I knew they were there because each inhalation brought her head down on her neck. Mistreating her and blaming her for it, her parents had convinced her that she was worthless. Venus had worked on these issues for decades before we met and has pretty much healed them since. Finding the history in her tissue and evicting it, however, was a relatively new experience for her, one she embraced wholeheartedly.

Her lung restrictions are fairly minor these days; therefore, her head and neck are much less affected by her breathing now than before. However, we recently found and released a lung restriction while trying to address some chronic arm and shoulder issues. A few days later, she awoke in the middle of the night and found herself breathing in a full, deep, and easy manner she couldn't recall having ever experienced before. During allergy season, she no longer needs medication and breathes like a champ.

Over the decades, Venus has established a very strong spiritual practice. She spends part of everyday surrendering ever deeper to who she really is. When she finds something at odds with her true nature, she lets it go. She readily admits that this isn't always easy, that she has bad days and feels down on occasion. When life serves her lemons, she makes lemonade and soldiers on. With introspection and self-acceptance, her physical, emotional, and spiritual health steadily improves. Her story reminds us that healing is spiritual work.

The Big C

If healing your personal trauma and finding your way "home" (spiritually) isn't reason enough to do emotional clearing work, here's another: cancer. Talk about your scariest symptom! Indeed, it is said that often the diagnosis can be as fatal as the disease because the shock, fear, and other afflictive emotions that arise on being told we have cancer can be overpowering. With cancer or any other life-threatening condition, we should immediately seek proper medical care, after which manual therapy can be an important adjunct.

It's common knowledge that cancer has many causes. The skyrocketing rates of cancer are probably largely attributable to increasing levels of stress and the proliferation of carcinogens, toxins, radiation, and electromagnetic pollution in our environment. For example, almost daily some chemist gins up a new carcinogen and puts it on the market where it finds its way into our air, water, food and homes. Currently, the state of California lists over 900 compounds as either carcinogenic or having reproductive or developmental toxicity. Genetic predispositions to certain types of cancer are well documented.

Traditional Chinese Medicine (TCM) has recognized the link between toxic emotions and cancer for 4,000 years. Subhuti Dharmananda, PhD, summarizes TCM's view in his paper "How Emotions May Contribute to Cancer" www. itmonline.org/arts/ cancemo.htm).

Some physicians even think that certain blood-types (A) are more prone to cancer (*Eat Right for Your Blood Type),* but few mention the role the emotions play. One wonders why? For at least the last 70 years, Western medicine has known that cancer is often linked to the emotions. Numerous American and European studies have shown that people who suppress emotions are more likely to end up with cancer. This personality type has been labeled C.

For example, in the 1950s all incoming medical students at Johns Hopkins School of Medicine were given personality tests and then tracked for two decades. A much higher percentage of those students who were unable or reluctant to express their feelings ended up with cancers than their Type A and Type B peers.

Type A's are the people who take life by the horns. Type B's have the "Easy come, easy go" attitude. Type C's tend to obsess over details, avoid conflict, have poorly developed boundaries, put themselves last, do not make friends easily, and stuff their feelings. Several of these traits suggest the possibility of relatively high levels of self-judgment and spiritual injury.

Much of this old information has been confirmed and better explained by recent advances in new medical subspecialties like psychoneuroimmunology. One would think this information about personality type would be publicized by physicians, especially oncologists, but it isn't.

However, at least one oncologist has made a study of the issues associated with various cancers. For ten years, Dr. Ryke-Geerd Hamer examined 20,000 cancer patients with all types of cancer. A German surgeon, Hamer wondered why cancer never seems to systematically spread directly from one organ to the surrounding tissue. He also noticed that all his cancer patients had had some kind of unresolved psycho-emotional conflict prior to the onset of their disease. When this emotional conflict was major and irreversible, for example the death of a loved one, the end of a career or important relationship, or some other personal or professional rejection, the cancer would usually appear in about two years. Based on what organ has cancer, he believes that he can predict with some reliability what the associated issue or emotion is.

In Dr. Hamer's research, X-rays showed a 'dark shadow' in exactly the same place in the brain for the same types of non-brain cancer. Dr. Hamer also found a 100% correlation between the location of the cancer in the body and the specific type of unresolved conflict. Based on these findings, Dr. Hamer suggested that unresolved conflicts lead to a gradual breakdown of the associated emotional reflex center in the brain. As a result, the brain starts sending misinformation to a specific organ, producing cancer cells in these same tissues. Dr. Hamer also suggested that metastases are not the same cancer spreading, but the result of new, associated conflicts, such as the very stress of having cancer or cancer treatment. Of course, this could explain why so many people never recover from being told that they have cancer.

Dr. Hamer found that when psychotherapy resolved the specific conflict, the cancer immediately stopped growing, the dark spot in the brain started to disappear, and healing edemas appeared around the damaged emotional center and the now-inactive cancer tissue. Eventually, the body encapsulated or eliminated the diseased tissue and replaced it with normal tissue.

Dr. Hamer developed a list showing the relationship between emotional issues and various target organs. He believed that cancer of the colon, for example, relates to ugly, indigestible conflict. These and other insights can be found at www. healingcancernaturally.com.

The foregoing information and anecdotes underscore the importance of having a healthy relationship with oneself and manual therapy's potential role in that. In thinking about the amazing outcomes I've seen, I'm reminded of two of my favorite Access Consciousness® affirmations. "How does it get any better than this?" "What else is possible?"

We should invoke these particular mantras anytime something good happens: in doing so, we're expressing both our gratitude for a gift bestowed and our willingness to receive even more. In my experience, the universe will respond positively.

CHAPTER 11

Troubleshooting

People often ask if manual therapy can address some chronic or mysterious challenge. Frequently, the answer is probably or yes. This chapter touches on nine categories of challenges common to many illnesses. The preceding chapters explain why these challenges respond to manual therapy.

Conventional medicine largely ignores mechanical restrictions and the emotions, even though they are usually factors in chronic challenges. Since manual therapy addresses both, it often succeeds where medicine has not, even for those who've almost given up hope. Moreover, unlike drugs, manual therapy almost always leaves the patient better off than before and that much closer to wellness.

Manual therapy, therefore, is always worth a shot. Since it has few negative side effects, we should consider it first, except in medical emergencies. Too often, we turn to it last, after drugs and other procedures have further compromised the body's systems.

Neil Nathan, MD, has spent decades specializing in treating tenacious health challenges. As a result, he has many insights into why patients don't get better and what can be done about it. Dr. Nathan places some of the blame on the lack of time many doctors spend with each patient. He believes that an hour is the minimum needed to understand what's really going on with a new patient. His systematic protocol, which includes manual therapy, eventually resolves most of his patients' chronic problems. Patients who can't seem to get well may want to read his book, *Healing Is Possible.*

One Off

While humans share the same general anatomy, the shape, position, and arrangement of internal organs and number of vertebrae and ribs can vary with the individual. Furthermore, each individual is unique, with her own constitution, genetic makeup, and history. These idiosyncrasies make the ability to use one's hands to find and correct problems in the tissues all the more critical. While manual therapists consider symptoms, history, and diagnoses, we treat where our hands are drawn.

Over the decades, my hands have found the following nine patterns again and again. While the first six appear to be largely mechanical, it's not that simple. Indeed, a mechanical restriction may be wholly emotional, spiritual, or psychological. Even when it's not, it can still be held in place by buried content. Here, then, are the most common issues I've found with chronic illness and pain:

1. Restrictions interfering with blood supply to the brain
2. Restrictions on other blood vessels and the heart
3. Restrictions on nerves and the brain
4. Lung restrictions
5. Stress
6. Restrictions compromising immune system function
7. Restrictions on internal organs

8. Being stuck in fight-or-flight: Reticular Activating System (RAS), Adverse Childhood Experiences (ACEs), Post Traumatic Stress Disorder (PTSD), and Complex Trauma.
9. Content: somatomized emotions, issues, beliefs, and attitudes.

Even when several of these situations occur in a single patient, treatment is relatively straightforward. Progress depends on the nature, extent, and number of illnesses and injuries and the patient's physical, mental, spiritual, and emotional health. Even patients who are seriously ill may progress quickly. While Attachment to Illness/Resistance to Health could easily be on this list, it is treated separately in the next chapter.

When we've already covered one of these challenges extensively, we've indicated so and kept the discussion here relatively brief. They are included here because of their importance and frequent occurrence.

1) Restrictions Interfering with Blood Supply to the Brain

The body's most important job is supplying the brain with oxygen, nutrients, and immune cells and removing metabolic wastes and toxins. This job requires adequate 1) deliveries of arterial blood to the cranium; 2) production and circulation of Cerebrospinal Fluid (CSF); and 3) drainage of venous blood and spent CSF from the cranium. (The associated vascular anatomy is presented in Chapter 1 as the ultimate example of the brilliance in the body's design.)

Four factors account for the brain's arterial shortfalls: 1) the convoluted bony pathways that the arteries must transit enroute; 2) the tendency of force to lodge in denser tissues like arteries; 3) the heaviness of heads relative to the strength of the neck; and 4) the abundance of mechanisms of injury: birth trauma, falls, and collisions. Sports and motor vehicles involve significant whiplash risks. No wonder so many of us have had multiple neck traumas.

Indications

Symptoms may appear anywhere in the body when the brain's blood supply is inadequate. This is true because the nervous system will short the rest of the body, with the exception of the heart, to minimize the brain's blood shortfall. Symptoms include weak cranial rhythms; headaches and migraines; skull rigidity; chronic neck and shoulder tension and musculoskeletal asymmetries; digestive challenges; cold extremities; and visual, hormonal, balance, diction, and cognitive challenges. After adequacy is restored to the brain, CSF circulation and CNS function usually improve and many of the symptoms will depart.

Discussion

Arterial insufficiency often goes undetected because doctors rarely check for it, except in extreme cases. Even then, it may not be the first thing that comes to mind. Indeed, a decade ago, newspapers reported a case where a man was stricken shortly after giving mouth-to-mouth resuscitation to his dog, which had been strangled in a trapper's snare. The man's symptoms had so baffled the doctors in Fairbanks, Alaska, that he was flown to Seattle. There, he stumped an even larger team of doctors at Harborview Hospital, the Pacific Northwest's largest trauma center, for several hours until someone thought to check the blood supply to his brain and found one carotid artery almost completely blocked (as a result of an old whiplash.)

Medicine may currently deem insignificant most arterial shortfalls, but tell that to a brain on short rations. Indeed, I've found this situation hundreds of times, and whenever I ask the patient's brain if it would like more blood, the brain's answer has always been an emphatic yes. Few of us would ever willingly choose suboptimal blood supply for our brain, yet many of my patients are experiencing just that, whether they realize it or not.

Chapter 3 described the importance of CSF. Vascular challenges, CSF deficiencies, and diseases of the mind may be linked. Studies suggest that CSF production diminishes by about 50% between the ages of 40 and 60. Certainly, this decrease plays a role in aging. By improving arterial supply and CSF production and circulation, manual therapy may delay the onset of CNS diseases such as Alzheimer's, Parkinson's, and dementia and reduce their severity.

If the brain's arterial supply is inadequate, CSF production and circulation will be sub-optimal. How could it be otherwise? CSF does not fall from the sky. Instead, this ultra-refined distillate comes from our arteries. The following story illustrates how this works, how easily it can be addressed, the interplay of content and restrictions, and consequences thereof.

In an idle moment between exercises on the last afternoon of a week's worth of Visceral Manipulation workshops, I asked a classmate at the next table how he was doing. It was a casual question. I had no inkling that he wasn't feeling well.

He: "Terrible! I've had a headache since I got here, and it's gotten worse with each passing day."

Thinking seven days was a long time for any headache, that he must be miserable, and his "Terrible!" might be an understatement, I said, "We have a few minutes. Would you like to work on it?"

He: "Yes."

As soon as he lay down on my table, I put my hands under the back of his head. It immediately rolled to the right. My first clue! Leaning close for privacy and to avoid disturbing classmates still practicing, I said, "Can we talk directly to your body for a minute? You okay with that?"

He: "Sure. Go ahead."

Me: "Ask your Circle of Willis if its blood supply is adequate?" (This structure is the brain's primary receiving terminal and distribution center for arterial blood.)

He: "No."

Me: "Circle of Willis, if the blood supply is better on one side than the other, which is better?"

He: "The left."

This confirmed my hunch. (The head usually tilts toward the side with the biggest arterial shortfall, in her case the right. This tilting shortens the distance between the heart and the more challenged side of the brain and reduces tension on the challenged artery, thereby reducing the shortfall as much as possible.)

Taking a guess, I put a finger on his right carotid artery. Immediately feeling my finger pulled upward, I followed the tension up through the skull, until the pull stopped.

Me: "Are you feeling this?"

He: "Yes."

Me: "We're just inside your cranium. I want to ask your body if this restriction we're working on right now is primarily physical, emotional, spiritual, or a combination?"

He: "Emotional." The blood flow through his carotid increased instantly.

Me: "Ask your body to show you what the primary emotion is."

He: "I know what it is: I always feel inadequate at these workshops. There are so many incredible therapists."

I knew exactly how he felt. Our instructor. Alain Croibier, DO, is Dr. Barral's primary collaborator, and Dr. Barral was teaching a different workshop in the next room. There must have been a dozen instructors and many of the best practitioners from around the world within 100 feet of us. One would have to have a very large ego, be an exceptional practitioner, or both not to feel otherwise.

But his answer surprised me because, until that moment, I'd always assumed that the body, given all its wisdom, would not dump content where it could most interfere with the brain's blood supply. Live and learn. Meanwhile, his arterial flow continued to improve.

Me: "Would it be okay, in theory, to let go of that sense of inadequacy?"

He: "Would it ever!"

Me: "Do it any way you want: exhale it; visualize letting go of it. You can replace it with its antithesis if you'd like: confidence, a sense of competency, adequacy. Whatever you like."

After a half a minute, I said, "I bet you're a good practitioner, aren't you?"

That upward pull on his carotid released as he said, "Yes, I do well by my patients."

By now, blood was flowing strongly and the artery's pulse had normalized. Without any prompting, his head moved to a neutral position, over his neck and shoulders. As this last was yet another clue that we had restored the blood flow in his right carotid sufficiently, I left his carotid and went back to cradling the back of his head in my palms.

"Wow," he said. "My headache is better."

"Good, because Alain is about to resume the lecture," I said. "Oh, and you now have a nice full cranial rhythm. No extra charge. Take it slow when you get up. You may be a little lightheaded."

He sat up, and feeling fine, slid off my table and into his seat as the lecture resumed. At most, this treatment had taken four minutes. Two hours later, his headache was almost completely gone.

Given more time, I would have asked him about previous whiplashes, when that sense of not being good enough began and where it came from, checked the three other arteries serving his brain, and rebalanced them all. In addition to emotional content like my colleague's, adhesions and scar tissue are often in play. In such cases, we work through them one at a time, starting with whichever exerts the strongest fascial pull or has the most constricted blood flow.

Restoring adequate arterial supplies to the brain is one of the most important services manual therapy can provide. Readers who've jumped ahead to this chapter can learn about the brain's arterial plumbing in Chapter 1 and, in Chapter 2, how we use the fascia to find and release restrictions anywhere in the body, including deep in the brain. Similarly, Chapter 9 explains why we are able to dialogue with tissues. The results speak for themselves.

Talking to tissues can be amazingly effective. Of course, we're really just releasing fascial restrictions, and we can do this silently, with our hands and intention, without any talking. However, when buried content is involved, dealing with it openly and directly, with the patient's conscious collaboration, validates the patient's experience, greatly expedites the process, and virtually eliminates the possibility of the restriction's return.

In the treatment just described, once the blood supply to the brain was restored, CSF production and circulation improved spontaneously, as evidenced by the stronger, fuller cranial rhythm. This is common. When this doesn't happen, there may be additional restrictions to find and release, including venous ones. After all, if the spent blood and CSF can't get out of the head, there's no room for the new arterial blood. We treat veins the same way we treat arteries.

In any event, a dramatically improved cranial rhythm is a good sign that we've succeeded. Patients often perceive the improvement in their CSF supply and circulation. The first time a colleague addressed a restriction on my vertebral artery, the sensations were unforgettable. I felt the blood snaking up multiple capillaries in my brain. I have no idea how many years the arterial tide had been out, but its return felt exquisite—I'm guessing akin to the relief intertidal creatures must feel when the tide finally returns after they've been drying in the sun and wind for hours.

2) Restrictions on Other Blood Vessels and the Heart

The brain may be the heart's most important customer, and the heart may be the CNS' most important supplier, but it's worth remembering that every organ and tissue in the body requires adequate circulation and nerve supply. That's why our body has 130,000 miles of blood vessels and 65,000 miles of nerves. Of course, so much plumbing and wiring present almost unlimited opportunities for mischief, which is why most of us have significant vascular (and neural) restrictions.

Chapter 1 described the body's hierarchical organization, wherein the heart and CNS share the top position. The previous section showed the effects of a restriction on a blood vessel serving the brain and how the body sacrifices muscles and the cervical vertebrae to minimize those effects. The body will go to equally great lengths to protect the heart from restrictions. This is because the heart is so important and even a small vascular restriction can interfere with it and significantly accelerate wear and tear, thanks to 72 beats per minute. (Chapter 1 described how post-surgical restrictions in the iliac veins (which return blood from the legs) were pulling a patient's heart backward and downward.)

The recruitment of less important structures to minimize the effect of arterial restrictions on the heart exacts a heavy price: it usually entails musculoskeletal imbalances, produces rigidity and pain, and may impede the vitality and function of other organs and tissues. This explains why releasing vascular restrictions can prevent or resolve a multitude of health challenges.

Indications

Muscle tension, joint pain, and reduced range of motion may be clues that there are restrictions on blood vessels. Many of these symptoms arise when the body draws an arm or leg inward toward the core or draws the head downward to reduce the tension on the heart resulting from a vascular restriction. When these are released, most patients immediately sense relief, sometimes profound. Rigidity or pain in the ribs or thoracic spine, shortness of breath, hypertension, rapid pulse, and circulatory challenges may be evidence of restrictions on the heart itself.

Discussion

Because of stress and the human tendency to take things personally, heart restrictions are quite common. When freeing them up, I always ask heart if its blood supply is adequate. Even in otherwise healthy patients, the answer is frequently "No." Whether that shortfall is emotional or physical or a combination, it's usually easily corrected. Ditto with restrictions on arteries in the extremities. Releasing those restrictions usually eliminates these otherwise troubling symptoms. Arguably, releasing restrictions on the heart and blood vessels are vitally important services manual therapy can perform for the body.

3) Restrictions on Nerves and the Brain

Like their vascular traveling companions, every inch of the 65,000 miles of nerves in the body has the potential to host a restriction that can impart a drag on the spinal cord and brain. Restrictions within the brain are also common. The latter result from collisions between the head and other objects, whiplashes, infections, and content.

Indications

The body will bend over backwards to minimize a neural restriction's drag on the CNS, thus creating all kinds of symptoms. Among the most common are joint and spinal challenges such as scoliosis, wry neck, dowager's hump, frozen shoulder, and headaches; back pain; palsies, sciatica, and numbness and tingling in the extremities; and cognitive challenges and problems with the special senses. Asymmetries in the head, face and cranial bones and their motions are often clues to restrictions within the brain itself.

Discussion

The nervous system began at conception as a single cell, growing outward from there like the trunk and roots of a tree from a single seed. As a result, peripheral nerves like to be stretched away from the core and brain. Most neural restrictions, including many of those in the CNS, lend themselves readily to manual therapy. For example, one patient complained of tingling and numbness in her right arm and hand. She came to see me after it had gotten to the point that she could barely lift and hold her coffee cup. We found and released a restriction on the median nerve at the wrist. That helped, but while stretching the median nerve from just above the wrist, we ran into another restriction in her shoulder. When I asked, she said that she'd injured her right shoulder in gymnastics in high school. Once we freed up some adhesions around the nerve junction (brachial plexus) on the right side of her neck, the tingling and weakness in her right arm stopped.

4) Lung Restrictions

The implications of lung restrictions were introduced in Chapter 4. Here, we explain why they are so common in the hope that readers take them more seriously. Healthy readers will be tempted to assume that they don't have lung restrictions. This is because most of us are unaware of having any. Explanations for this lack of awareness include: the gradual onset of symptoms, obscuration by more attention-getting symptoms; and the tendency to quickly get used to something that occurs so frequently (17,000 or more inhalations per day). As a result, compromised breathing frequently becomes the new normal within an hour or two.

Indications

Symptoms of lung restrictions include spinal challenges such as vertebral fractures, bone spurs, degeneration and arthritis; shortness of breath and labored, shallow, and neck breathing; shoulder and hip challenges; hernias; high blood pressure and other heart challenges; immune and digestive challenges; and fascial armoring—thickened bands of fascia around the respiratory diaphragm. Lung restrictions interfere with heart mobility and motility and make the heart work harder. They can result in compressing the brainstem and cerebellum. The variety and distribution of impacts results from the importance of adequate gas exchange and the large movements required to accomplish it.

Discussion

Rather than ask if we have lung restrictions, the more relevant question is how many do we have and how significant are they? The ubiquity of lung restrictions stems from many factors, beginning with the number and variety of possible causes: respiratory infections; aspiration of liquids; inhalation of pollutants; vaccinations; and physical, chemical, thermal and emotional trauma.

Indeed, consider chemical exposures. Most of us are constantly barraged by particulates and vapors, including baby powder, dust, ash, pollen, smoke, soot, sawdust, fuels, solvents, cleansers, adhesives, air fresheners, perfumes, deodorants, hair sprays, cooking sprays, magic markers, outgassing building products like particle board, adhesives, paints and stains, synthetic fabrics, vehicular emissions, pesticides, herbicides, fungicides, compressed gasses, and so forth. The possibilities are nearly as endless as they are ubiquitous and unavoidable. Because breathing is not optional, the assault is nearly continuous, the effects cumulative.

The sheer volume of gas our lungs exchange is another important factor. At rest, adult males move about ten quarts of air per minute while resting and between 50 and 60 quarts per minute while running slowly. (Females a little less.) This can add up to between 2000 and 4000 gallons during a lazy day, while an athlete might inhale 900 gallons or air during a single hour of heavy exercise. The lungs' internal surfaces amount to 1000 square feet, about half a tennis court, affording ample opportunities for restrictions. The complexity of the lungs themselves presents another factor: the miles of air passages, the sheer number of alveoli, and so forth. Restrictions are also common in the dividers (septa or fissures) that compartmentalize the lungs into lobes (upper, middle, and lower) and in the connective tissues (pleura) that separate the lungs from the thoracic cavity.

The lungs undergo larger continuous volumetric changes than any other internal organ. With 6.3 million inhalations a year, those changes make lung restrictions the body's most important generators of repetitive motion injuries. The frequency and volumes explain why lung restrictions have such widespread and serious impacts. Furthermore, the associated compressive forces strengthen over time as the vertebrae and its support systems weaken. In other words, as the damage accumulates, it also accelerates.

Normally, the heart swings back and forth across the thorax six to eight times per minute. Lung restrictions interfere with these movements, impede the heart's beating, and make it work that much harder. Instead of the continuous massage the heart would have received absent lung restrictions, in their presence the heart experiences around-the-clock buffeting. The body minimizes those effects by shallow breathing and tightening lumbar, thoracic, and cervical muscles. Unfortunately, this denies our cells their full ration of oxygen and produces musculoskeletal imbalances and pain.

Chapter 3 described how a habit of deep breathing in the presence of a large lung restriction tore one patient's descending colon from its hanger under the spleen, resulting in a bowel obstruction. That story underscored the power of the lungs and their ability to cause problems.

The lungs also play another important, if generally unrecognized role: the partial vacuum in the lungs that facilitates inhalation also provides substantial lift to our abdominal organs. For example, the liver is our heaviest internal organ; the average adult's weighs about seven pounds. In a living person, however, thanks to that lift, the effective weight of the same liver is essentially half that, or about 3.5 pounds.

This lift diminishes with distance from the respiratory diaphragm; therefore, the stomach, spleen, and transverse colon are the other primary beneficiaries. However, the rest of the colon, small intestine, pancreas, kidneys, bladder, and uterus benefit from having less weight bearing down on them. However, if lung restrictions diminish the pressure differential across the diaphragm, all the viscera in the lower abdomen will find themselves shouldering increasing weight from above, diminishing their mobility, motility, function, and vitality.

The structural design of our thorax accounts for much of the connection between physical trauma and lung restrictions. Our ribs transmit impacts from falls and collisions to the front of our thorax. In many ways, this is fortunate because the articulations between sternum and ribs are essentially double jointed: rib end-joint-cartilage-joint-sternum. This cartilaginous spacer between each rib and the sternum allows for considerable accommodation—especially compared to the situation at the back where the joints between the ribs and vertebrae have almost no room to spare. A fall or even moving one's arm can trap a rib out of joint with the vertebrae, producing muscle spasms and nearly intolerable pain for days. However, restrictions between the ribs and sternum exact a price, too: they can jam the sternum so that it interferes with the heart, inhalation, and the immune system.

Impacts from seatbelts and airbags are another common source of lung trauma and restrictions. While the rib cage and thoracic spine offer bony protection, they also can become mechanisms of injury, transmitting the energy of an impact to the lungs and associated blood vessels. A broken rib may puncture the lung and collapse it.

The left lung has an upper and lower lobe; the right, an upper, middle, and lower. In the presence of restrictions, one or more of these lobes won't be inflating properly. The restriction could be within a lobe; on a fissure between lobes; on the diaphragm, pleura, or mediastinum; or an adjacent rib, vertebrae, or sternum. A chimney-like fascial structure running from the base of our neck to our respiratory diaphragm, the mediastinum separates the right and left lung, creating a virtual space for our esophagus and pericardium/ heart.

Given all of the above, lung restrictions are often the first thing I notice when I cradle a patient's head in my palms. I've felt them from just about everywhere else on the body: in the chest and on the legs, feet, and arms. They can even be visible in the movement of a patient's clothing.

Of course, there are several other common sources of breathing challenges: stress, being stuck in fight-or-flight, and emotional armoring. We'll consider stress next.

5) Stress

In discussing the significance of lung restrictions, we would be remiss if we overlooked the relationship between the respiratory diaphragm and stress. Often, we shrug off stress as if it entailed no health consequences or there was nothing that we could do about it, even though doctors often refer to stress as the silent killer.

Indications

A partial list of symptoms includes: shallow, rapid breathing; back pain; elevated blood pressure, rapid heartbeat; hypertension; muscle tension; clenched jaw, grinding teeth; fatigue, chronic fatigue, adrenal exhaustion; concentration, hearing, digestive, immune, sexual, and sleep challenges; depression, low self-esteem, excessive worrying, anxiety; obesity. For a complete list, try googling *www.webmd.com*.

Discussion

Patients who exhibit any of the symptoms or have been under prolonged stress may be stuck in the stress reflex, which was described in the previous chapter. Freeing up their diaphragm and teaching them how to turn the reflex off and relax their diaphragm may resolve their health issues and prevent or slow spinal challenges.

Thanks to this reflex, which develops when we are about six-months old, most of us hold tension in our respiratory diaphragm. (We described the mechanical implications of the stress reflex and how it sabotaged one runner's Mount Marathon race in the previous chapter.) By definition, all reflexes are automatic and non-conscious.

The stress reflex is most obvious in toddlers and young children because they haven't learned how to conceal it. When stressed, in addition to tightening the respiratory diaphragm, they will hold their breath, make fists, scrunch the front of their bodies, bring their knees toward their chests, and turn red or purple while crying or screaming.

With age, most of us get better at hiding the outward expressions of this reflex, but not the diaphragmatic tightening and its attendant physiological consequences. The diaphragm doesn't automatically relax after the stress ends; instead, the tension tends to remain and increase with each subsequent episode, again without our awareness. Fortunately, mindfulness (meditation), yoga, physical exercise, or even simple breathing exercises can reverse the process. However, when the stressor persists for weeks or months, say in the case of health, financial, professional, or relationship problems, getting the tissues to relax completely may require serious, concerted effort. For an easy exercise to relax the diaphragm, please see Appendix A.

6) Restrictions Compromising Immune Function

We've just mentioned that lung restrictions and stress can interfere with our immune system's phenomenal abilities, which were described in Chapter 3. To summarize, the immune system can track down, destroy, and remove pathogens; clean up adhesions and restrictions; clear out arteries; and repair or replace any damaged tissue in the body (with stem cells). A small gland located between the sternum and the heart, the thymus, governs immune activities and provides our access to the system.

Indications

Common symptoms include frequent colds and flus, chronic infections, wounds that are slow to heal, allergies, and autoimmune challenges.

Discussion

Compromised immune systems typically result from one or more of the following:

- Restrictions on thymus' more important, neighboring structures such as the heart, brain, and lungs
- Content: thymus' neighborhood is a favorite dumping ground for emotional overloads
- Exposures to immune suppressing aerosols, gasses, liquids, and solids
- Electromagnetic radiation (computer screens and cell phones)

This list goes a long way towards explaining the epidemic of immune challenges.

Location, location, location is fine in real estate, but living next door to the heart, lungs, and aorta, some of the body's most important organs, does not work to thymus's advantage because of the extent to which thymus's needs are sacrificed for the benefit of its neighbors.

Indeed, our bodies are designed to protect the heart from physical trauma. When we fall, this design focuses forces onto the sternum, leaving thymus in the proverbial "between a rock (heart) and a hard place (sternum)." Another critical priority, delivering adequate blood to the brain, often results in upward tension on the heart, again compressing thymus between the heart and sternum. Finally, the heart and lungs are favorite dumping grounds for emotional upsets, which also crowd thymus and compromise its functioning.

Most of us ignore our immune system when we are well and fault it when we are ill—precisely when we should be helping, not criticizing, our immune system. The immune system isn't lazy or stupid: with a little love in the form of space and energy, it works miracles.

When someone has an infection, cold, flu, pneumonia, immune challenge, adhesion or scar tissue on a critical structure, or even inadequate blood supply to the heart, the thymus gland will be the first structure I work with. We always address thymus' needs for energy first, before enlisting its assistance, so that we can tap the immune system's full power. Thanks to the body's hierarchical nature, we may have to focus on the lungs, heart, and brain for several treatments before we can address thymus' other needs (space and blood). Nonetheless, thymus will still work remarkably well if we've satisfied its energy needs.

Our tendency to blame our immune system when we are sick is doubly unfortunate because it's probably working hard under some sort of handicap and deserves gratitude and support rather than criticism. For example, with allergies and autoimmune challenges, it's usually been thrown a curve. Many allergies begin when we experience an emotional overload in the presence of an otherwise benign substance. It seems that the nervous and immune systems have conflated the substance with the afflictive emotions and stored this information for future reference. When that substance reenters the person's energy field, the nervous system equates it with the earlier threat and initiates an allergic response.

In this sense, an allergy resembles an anxiety or panic attack, with all the attendant chemical changes. For example, I had one young patient with a nut allergy. We learned that it all had begun seven years earlier. She was eating a Nutella (hazelnut spread) and jelly sandwich for lunch when her parents resumed one of their frequent and bitter arguments. Rather than protest, she swallowed her feelings (fear, anger, concern, frustration, resentment) and perhaps some of her parents' feelings, along with the Nutella. This comingling of feelings and substance resulted in a sensitivity to hazelnuts that rapidly blossomed into a full-blown allergy and eventually encompassed all nut products.

Of course, somatomization—storing emotional overloads in the tissues—is automatic and subconscious. Therefore, we're usually unaware that this material is parked in our tissues. But in the safety of a treatment, the patient remembered the fight that led to her allergy. From there, she was able to let go of the emotions, change the energy in the affected organs, and ask the immune system to dial back its response to the allergen, thus eliminating the allergy.

Allergic reactions that trigger anaphylactic shock are life-threatening. The airway contracts, leading to asphyxia and cardiac arrest. Absent immediate medical intervention, death may occur within minutes, even in otherwise healthy persons. Medical approaches to allergies typically amount to management rather than elimination; tend to be expensive; and involve unwanted side effects. In contrast, when people are not in the middle of a life-threatening allergic response, manual therapy can make light work of allergies as the following story suggests:

"Gina" came to me for help with chronic pain in her lower back and a history of allergies. An exposure to dog dander could send her into anaphylactic shock. She carried an "epi" (epinephrine) pen with her at all times to improve her chances of reaching the emergency room before her heart stopped. Over the decades, she'd endured many trips to the ER and all kinds of allergy treatments to no avail.

After releasing some restrictions behind her kidneys, we still had a few minutes left. I asked her if she wanted to tackle her allergy. She did.

Hearing the answers to the questions I ask patients helps me formulate the next question, but is usually not necessary. What is critical is that patients allow themselves to hear the answers. As we'd just met, barely knew each other and had only a few minutes, I didn't want her wasting precious seconds weighing the pros and cons of sharing something personal with me. Therefore, I told her that she needn't share any of the answers with me; she just needed to be willing to hear them herself.

The process was simple. It went like this:

Me: "Ask your body to show you the very first time you developed a sensitivity to dogs."

Fifteen seconds later, she: "Okay, got it."

Me: "Is the organ most affected the lungs?"

She, immediately: "Correct."

Me: "Ask your body what emotion, issue, belief, or attitude is related to the allergy."

She: "Okay. Got it."

Me: "Are you ready to let go of that today?"

She: "Yes."

Me: "Great. Do it anyway you like: with a visualization, with the breath. You could just exhale it. Do you want to replace it with anything? Its antithesis? Some peace, acceptance, self-compassion, self-love?"

She: "I'm on it."

Me: "Gina's lungs, are there any other emotions, issues, beliefs or attitudes associated with this dog allergy?"

She: "Yes."

Me: "Yours or some other guy's?"

She: "Both."

Me: "Are you willing to let go of all that?"

She: "Yes."

Me: "You know the drill."

She: "On it."

Me: "Lungs, would you like some energy today?"

She: "Oh, would I!"

Me: "If the energy came in the form of light, what color or colors would be most helpful?"

She: "Pink."

Me: "Okay. Visualize a beautiful beam of pink light flooding your lungs. Changing their energy. Under new management."

She: "Got it."

Me: "Gina's thymus, can you recognize dog dander when it comes into Gina's energy field?"

She: "Of course."

Me: "Would it be okay to dial back the response when it does in the future?"

She: "Sure."

Me: "Thymus, would you like some energy today? If so,—"

She, cutting me off: "Sure. White light."

Me: "All the colors of the visible spectrum. The rainbow. An energy smorgasbord. Go for it. If the color should change, go with that. I'm afraid we're out of time. Thank you, Gina. Thank you, Gina's thymus. Thank you, lungs."

Shortly after that treatment, I left town for two weeks. When I bumped into Gina on my first day back, she was excited to see me. Pulling out her smartphone, she showed me a picture of her petting a dog. Having forgotten all about her allergy, I had no idea what I was supposed to be seeing, or why.

Gina explained, "At first, I didn't see how we could've cured my allergy so quickly but after a few days, I got curious and decided to do a little experiment. I called a friend who owned a dog, and with my epi pen close at hand, and a car and driver ready to whisk me to the ER just in case, I bent down and started patting the dog. For about five minutes. When that failed to trigger an allergic response, I rubbed the dog, hugged it, and basically loved it up one side and down the other. For about ten minutes. No allergic response. No anaphylactic shock. No epi pen or trip to the ER. I'm still amazed. You're a star!" She gave me a big hug.

"Well, thanks, but so are you and your thymus," I said. "I've never seen anyone eliminate an allergy so fast. We should put you in Guinness."

"My boyfriend and I are talking about getting a dog. I've always loved them."

In less than ten minutes, Gina had managed to discover and release the emotions at the root of her canine allergy and then, working with her thymus gland, lungs, and nervous system, eliminated it. Subsequently, she bought a dog and has had no further sensitivity.

While delighted, I wasn't surprised. Her treatment had been based on Dr. Upledger's pioneering work with the immune system. I merely followed his protocol. These and many other results suggest that he was correct: allergies and other immune and auto-immune problems need not be the lifelong sentences that so many people assume they are.

With allergies, most of us assume that the immune system is mistaken or malfunctioning. Dr. Upledger believed otherwise, intuiting that the immune system was viewing an otherwise benign substance as a threat thanks to its association with a previous emotional trauma. Since a primary task is protecting us from pathogens, we should expect the immune system to react strongly to substances that the nervous system equates with danger.

A similar approach holds great promise for the treatment of autoimmune disorders. When there is an autoimmune challenge, for example, arthritis, buried content may be the culprit. This possibility should be fully explored and exhausted. If the patient can find out when the problem began, what was going on at the time, and release the somatomized emotions, the patient should be able to stop the body from attacking itself.

Although immune challenges are on the rise, it doesn't necessarily follow that immune systems are increasingly malfunctioning. They are under unprecedented assault from stress and environmental pollutants. However, for any given autoimmune challenge, there probably is something foreign in our tissues, someone else's energy or content that varies from our essential nature. A good initial approach to resolving immune problems might be to collaborate with the system, rather than criticize or wage war against it.

7) Restrictions on Internal Organs

Since the significance of restrictions on internal organs has already been discussed at length, what follows is a summary of the importance of visceral mobility and motility, which was fully explained in Chapter 3.

Indications

Symptoms of organ restrictions include pain, spinal issues, and organ-specific and systemic challenges, such as digestive, circulatory, endocrine, cognitive, reproductive, or musculoskeletal challenges. In other words, practically anything. Indeed, restrictions on internal organs are exceedingly common and account for between 50 and 60% of all spinal problems that Dr. Barral has treated.

Discussion

Any restriction that impedes the motion of any organ or interferes with the organ's blood supply or energy will eventually have significant health consequences. Restrictions on and in internal organs result from infections; surgeries; and thermal, electrical, chemical, physical, emotional, and spiritual trauma. All organs need adequate space, blood, mobility, motility, and energy, while CNS organs also need adequate CSF. When we address these basic needs, many health challenges disappear.

In addition to the restrictions on nerves, arteries, and the heart and lungs which were discussed earlier in this chapter, restrictions are also common on the abdominal organs and endocrine glands. For example, Chapter 3 described the various ways one could end up with a restriction on the stomach and Chapter 10 discussed thyroid restrictions.

Restrictions between the colon and the abdominal wall are very common and can produce irregularity and major hip challenges. We can visualize the potential consequences of a colon restriction if we think of the lumbar spine as a ship's mast and the ascending colon on one side and the descending on the other as stays. On a properly tuned mast, the tension on each stay will be balanced, the mast straight. The ascending colon hangs off the liver, the descending off the spleen. Running between the two, the transverse colon hangs like a loosely furled sail, communicating any tensions from one side to the other. If one side of the colon has a restriction on it and is tighter than the other, the spine will eventually bend toward the tighter side, compressing the discs on that concave side and inviting them to pop out on the convex side opposite. This is just one way a colon restriction might produce back pain and spinal problems or interfere with liver, spleen, or kidney function.

At the same time, a large colon restriction is likely to approximate the hip to the ribs on that side. We often see one hip "hiked" or higher than the other and rotated in or out and forward or backward. (This is frequently attributed to a tight quadratus lumborum (QL) muscle also known as the hip-hiker muscle. However, more often than not, the QL has been recruited to compensate for an underlying restriction on the colon, kidney, or some other internal organ.) The asymmetry in the hips and shoulders may be more obvious when a person is standing up or lying on their back. Imagine what this twist might do to the lumbar vertebrae and the joint between the sacrum and hip (sacroiliac joint) over time. Untreated, the resultant skewed mechanics probably account for a significant percentage of the hip replacements and lumbar fusions that are now so common.

On the other hand, when both sides of the colon have restrictions, it's common to have almost no space between the lowest ribs and the hips, a sign that the lumbar spine is being compressed. Eventually, this will produce serious back problems. Meanwhile, the all-important kidneys are trapped in a difficult space. Their mobility and motility and function will be impaired, and we may experience that as back pain, low energy, and bladder problems.

Speaking of function, the colon moves fecal matter by peristalsis, essentially "doing the wave." Anywhere there is a restriction, the "wave" will pretty much come to a dead stop, only to have to restart once beyond. Anyone who has ever trapped a jump-rope or garden hose under a piece of furniture understands the problem. Restoring the wave will require energy and effort, and the wave will not recover its former vitality for some distance, if ever. This is how a colon restriction could result in sluggish digestion, irregularity, Irritable Bowel Syndrome, perhaps even diverticulitis. Considering irregularity alone, a colon with a large restriction might vacillate between constipation and loose stools, the latter being an effective if inconvenient strategy to move things along.

Obviously, colon restrictions could affect the liver and spleen through their direct connections (fascial hangers called flexures), but those aren't the colon's only connections to neighboring structures. In Chapter 3, we mentioned the greater omentum, which hangs off the bottom of the stomach and first part of the duodenum (small intestine). The omentum attaches directly to the ascending, transverse, descending and sigmoid colons and carries much of the colon's nerve and blood supply. Therefore, a colon restriction might also affect the small intestine, stomach, heart, or CNS, in addition to spleen and liver.

Motility with the colon consists of the ascending and descending moving in sync with each other. In other words, both move simultaneously up, out, and back in *inspir*, and in, down, and forward in *expir*. Moreover, the small intestine follows and mimics the descending as if they were the two components of a gear. We can imagine how a restriction on either would impede the motility of the other.

Most of us probably have at least one significant restriction on our colon, more if we've had a traumatic childhood, done contact sports, been in fights, had car wrecks (seatbelt/air bag injuries), or had our wind knocked out. All of the above suggests why, in many cases of digestive challenges, freeing up the restrictions might be a more efficacious approach than treating the symptoms with medication or spinal manipulation alone.

As we explained in Chapter 1, since the body is hierarchical and intelligent, it often recruits and sacrifices less important structures to protect more important ones. Therefore, in looking for the root of a problem, it's always worth checking up the hierarchical ladder. For example, many chronic musculoskeletal problems that have not responded quickly to massage or chiropractic may be symptoms of a mechanical restriction on a deeper, more important structure such as an artery, nerve, or internal organ.

Similarly, when the body has recruited muscles and bones to minimize the effect of a restriction on an internal organ, massaging those muscles and manipulating the spine will likely undercut the body's best efforts to protect the more important structure, no matter how well intentioned and gifted the practitioner. Furthermore, releases on structures that have been recruited are not likely to last. Better to find and treat the underlying restriction. Then the musculoskeletal packaging will return to its day job, with little or no additional help.

Often, finding and releasing restrictions on internal organs resolves challenges quickly and improves prognoses. Since mechanical restrictions are ubiquitous, the solution to a stubborn health challenge may be buried somewhere in this haystack.

8) Fight-or-Flight: RAS, ACEs, PTSD, and Complex Trauma

Earlier in this chapter, we discussed the relationship between stress and the respiratory diaphragm. Because the nervous system monitors every activity in out body, a tight diaphragm can keep us stuck in fight-or-flight. This section presents a review of how previous physical and emotional trauma can keep us stuck in fight-or-flight, often for years. In mild cases, we may be unaware of the problem, even though we may be aware of the symptoms.

Chapter 6 introduced the Reticular Activating or Reticular Alarm System (RAS), the subsystem of the CNS most intimately involved with survival. The RAS involves five structures in the brain (cerebellum, medulla oblongata, pons, amygdala, and the hippocampus) and the adrenal cortices atop each kidney.

Humans and other mammals are hard-wired to make one of four responses to danger: fight, flight (run), flop, or freeze. Though usually overlooked and unmentioned, the last two options sometimes work when all seems lost. Flop is essentially going limp, as when one faints, and can make it awkward for a predator to move us. Freeze is perhaps most famously exercised by possums whose stiffness and stillness often fools predators looking for a fresh meal.

We'll focus on the two most common responses, fight or flight. Typically, if we fight or flee successfully, the system resets itself. However, if we are unable to fight or flee and the danger or threat persists, we're likely to become stuck in elevated alert. This has enormous physiological consequences: for starters, a significant share of the oxygen and nutrients normally destined for the higher brain centers are diverted to the RAS structures at the expense of those higher centers.

Indications

Symptoms of being stuck in fight-or-flight include chronic muscular tension; digestive, cognitive, sleep, and immune challenges; anxiety, adrenal fatigue and exhaustion; and a tendency toward passivity or aggression. In addition to all that, PTSD often makes it difficult to distinguish present reality from past events. Flashbacks and other extreme emotional and mental disturbances are common.

Discussion

While any of the above may be signs that RAS is elevated, any chronic challenge may be a clue. Indeed, when questioned, almost every patient from one naturopathic clinic because of chronic digestive challenges reported that their RAS was stuck near or beyond the top of the scale. Neither patients nor naturopaths had been aware of this, though it turned out to be the root of their problem.

Ironically, having a chronically elevated RAS is in itself a danger because when we are stuck on high alert, the RAS is trying to monitor 50 times more neural traffic than it was designed for. This can delay detection of danger, and the already tight muscles and associated adrenalin shortage virtually guarantee a sub-optimal response.

Situations that elevate RAS are exceedingly common. They include exposure to physical or emotional danger in all their forms when we are unable to fight or flee. Occurring from conception onward, these situations aren't just limited to combat or hazardous jobs, but arise when we have an unmanageable workload or abusive associates from whom we can't escape. These could be family members, caregivers, teachers, neighbors, coworkers, and supervisors. These almost endless possibilities explain why elevated-RASs are at epidemic levels, even in relatively safe parts of the relatively safe United States and Canada.

The good news is that identifying a RAS problem and effecting a reset is relatively easy. We simply ask the patient's body where their RAS is set on a scale of 1 to 100, without telling them what is normal. If the answer suggests that RAS is set too high or too low, we ask the patient's body if a reset would be in the patient's best interest. If the answer is "yes" and the patient gives his body permission, the reset begins. They usually complete on their own, often in minutes, but occasionally take a day or two.

After an RAS reset, the affected systems usually improve automatically and quickly. We end up calmer, better able to concentrate and use our higher brain functions. Our immune and digestive systems work better. Paradoxically, we are safer: no longer trying to examine every nerve impulse, the cerebellum, medulla, and pons are likely to recognize danger sooner. Our relaxed muscles are more capable of responding and have a full reservoir of adrenaline for fueling the response.

Occasionally, a situation or upset will re-elevate RAS. Such cases may require several resets over a period of weeks or months to stabilize RAS at a healthier level. Occasionally a patient will report an exceptionally low RAS. While rare, this is just another strategy for dealing with chronic stress or danger. Treatment remains basically the same as with an elevated RAS.

The Proof is in the Purring

In addition to improving the immune, digestive, cognitive, energy, and musculoskeletal problems associated with elevated RASs, patients who have had their RAS reset report experiencing a profound sense of calm, dramatically increased resistance to previous irritations, and the ability to relax and enjoy life in ways previously impossible. For example, one of my patients told me that she loved her grandkids but their jumping up and down on her sofa, shrieking joyfully, and spilling soda was driving her nuts. It turned out her RAS had been very high for decades. Three weeks later, when she returned for another session, I asked her how things were going. She said that she really enjoyed her grandkids' last visit. When I asked why, she said she'd been jumping up and down on the sofa with them and making just as much noise as they were.

When we get objective feedback about manual therapy, it bears mention, even if it's anecdotal. Another patient had taken in a stray cat. She said the cat loved to be petted but was skittish and refused to lie on her lap. Hearing this made me curious about the patient's RAS. When we discovered that it was significantly elevated, we did a reset. Once she was home, the moment she sat down on her sofa, the cat climbed onto her lap, curled up, began to purr, and went to sleep. Apparently, the cat perceived a change in her mistress' energy field sufficient enough to finally feel safe.

PTSD

Once thought to be limited mostly to combat survivors and emergency responders, PTSD can affect anyone who has been exposed to or witnessed overwhelming trauma, including children. Someone who has been through a serious car accident can get PTSD. Manual therapy can also be a useful component of the more comprehensive approach required for successfully treating PTSD.

Huge progress has been made in the diagnosis and treatment of all kinds of PTSD in the past few decades. Those interested in PTSD should read *Waking the Tiger* by Peter A. Levine. For more than a decade, the larger psychiatric community stubbornly resisted the notion that childhood PTSD differed from that which occurs in adults, but the experts treating kids eventually prevailed, and we now have a separate diagnosis. This is important because untreated childhood PTSD produces severe developmental and adaptive challenges. There are several effective treatments for childhood PTSD. For those interested in this topic, a must read is *The Body Keeps the Score*, by Bessel A. van der Kolk, MD.

While PTSD can arise from a single, overwhelming experience such as a car accident with serious injuries, a hostage situation, or a shooting, Complex Trauma tends to stem from repetitive traumas, particularly in childhood. For example, if a child is repeatedly traumatized every couple of months for several years, the repetition could burnish in the trauma and resultant sense of fear, powerlessness, and victimhood. Complex Trauma is a relatively new diagnosis but one which may be helpful in understanding why some patients are slow to respond to treatment and, more importantly, in improving their outcomes.

In the last decade, again after much resistance, the medical community has also come to recognize a closely-related syndrome: Adverse Childhood Experiences (ACEs). Ten common risk factors have been identified. These include exposure to physical violence, frequent verbal abuse, inappropriate touching or sexual behavior, feeling unloved, not having enough to eat or drink, having separated or divorced parents, living with someone depressed or mentally ill, exposure to someone abusing drugs or alcohol, having a family member incarcerated, living in a dangerous area. Children who experience three or more of these situations will not develop normal resilience to life's challenges and are much more likely to experience scholastic challenges, become truants, abuse drugs and alcohol, drop out of school, engage in criminal activities, and experience serious health challenges by their thirties, including heart disease.

ACEs are both a public and personal health challenge. Fortunately, they respond readily to treatment. Communities that have tackled ACEs have seen dramatic reductions in scholastic and behavioral challenges and criminal activity. A simple Google search will pull up the Center for Disease Control's ACE questionnaire. The film *Resilience* provides a great summary of the syndrome, its treatment, and successful outcomes.

Given all the ethnic, national, and racial strife around the world, RAS, PTSD, Complex Trauma, and ACEs probably constitute some of the planet's most significant health challenges, in part because of the damage they cause to individual sufferers, and in part because of the endless cycles of violence and retaliation they spawn, engulfing communities, nations and entire regions in wars, ethnic cleansing and genocide.

9) Buried Content

It's no accident that many of the anecdotes in this book involve somatomized emotions, issues, beliefs, and attitudes because that's how our bodies deal with overloads. Some readers will balk at the suggestion that their challenge might be partly emotional or spiritual. However, it's important to remember that no matter how well we know our story, we have no idea what our brain has parked in our tissues until we find it. The idea that a given challenge might largely stem from somatomized overloads should be good news because emotional trauma is usually easy to find and release. (Chapter 8 describes what content is, how it gets somatomized, and what it does then.) In addition to creating or maintaining mechanical restrictions, the content communicates continuously with our CNS, keeping us stuck in some degree of fight-or-flight.

Content creates and maintains illness and renders us injury-prone, especially when it involves damage to our relationship with ourselves. Discussed in Chapter 9, these spiritual injuries carry implicit messages that we deserve illness and injuries and that we don't deserve to be well. If your inclination is to assume that such messages can't be part of your problem, I urge you to read or reread Chapters 8 and 9. Often beginning as childhood survival strategies, these messages can be subtle and tenacious, but their consequences are ruinous. Manual therapy can help us find, eliminate, and replace them with healthier beliefs and attitudes.

Indications

Any health challenge may be a symptom that somatomized content is making mischief in our tissues. Any challenge that hasn't responded to medicine probably has a mechanical component, namely a restriction. Stubborn restrictions that don't respond readily to purely manual approaches often involve content. Earlier in this chapter, we discussed the effects of stress. Later, we explained how the RAS can get stuck in an elevated alert mode. Somatomized content is a third avenue that can keep us stuck in fight or flight. It's probably the most common too. Content can create illness and injuries; produce chronic pain; and lead to adrenal fatigue, adrenal exhaustion, chronic fatigue, anxiety, and digestive, endocrine, and immune and autoimmune challenges.

Discussion

Indeed, the more vehemently patients insist that their challenge is purely physical, the more likely it isn't. In fact, the vehemence itself is often a clue. Typically, that's our ego speaking, struggling to maintain control, even at the cost of keeping us sick. Since somatomization is unconscious and automatic, we usually can't know that we've somatomized something until we find it. Unexplained, mysterious, or chronic symptoms may be a sign that we should look under the hood. Fear not. Most of our buried content is no longer of consequence, were it not for the pathology it engenders.

Whether we realize it or not, most of us have been emotionally or spiritually wounded. Often. This is not necessarily a reflection on us or anyone else, but a fact of life. Humans are sensitive beings. The more an individual pretends otherwise, the more likely he's been deeply hurt. Even if our childhood was completely normal, we'll still have somatomized content in our tissues. In any event, the upshot can be chronic pain and health challenges. As Chapters 9 and 10 show, the good news is that manual therapy can help address that too. What's done is done. We can't change our history, but we can find where it is parked in the tissues and defang it so that we can move on.

It is worth repeating that dumping the overload in our tissue is an unconscious, hard-wired, and automatic survival strategy and CNS service. We wouldn't want it any other way when we are actually in danger. However, often when we somatomize content, we aren't in actual physical danger. We may simply be busy, emotionally vulnerable, or in a situation not conducive to our processing the emotion or experience or expressing how we feel. Weeks or years later, we're usually more capable of releasing the associated content.

Unfortunately, by the time we are safe again, we've either forgotten the emotional overload or don't realize we've dumped it in our tissues. Even if the situation around the overload becomes one of those stories that we replay over and over in our heads, and even if we suspect that we've somatomized some content, we won't know where to look for it, although existing restrictions, concurrent or recent injury sites, and organs with chronic challenges are likely suspects. A restriction that doesn't respond readily to manual therapy may be a clue that some history or content—an emotion, belief, attitude, or issue—is involved.

For several reasons, working with old content rarely results in re-traumatization. In hindsight, most stored content is trifling, even if it was very significant once. This change often stems from our having grown emotionally, built a sturdier base of support, or worked on it in our minds. Furthermore, the same survival instincts that stuffed the content into the tissues in the first place will prevent its rediscovery and release if we are still not safe or are not yet equipped to handle the content, memories, and associated feelings.

But, conscious or otherwise, the fear of re-traumatization can impede our letting go of restrictions and healing. When this is so, the way forward is information, education, and manual therapists who are comfortable with emotional release work and can provide the necessary safety and support.

Though we are not consciously aware of the emotional overloads parked in our tissues, they communicate continuously with our brain, leaving us in a state of alertness, leaving us even more vulnerable to everyday stress. Finding and evicting the somatomized content is one of several effective manual techniques for addressing those problems.

Chapter 3 described a patient whose blood sugar levels were dangerously high because of emotions parked around his bile duct, putting his sphincter of Oddi in spasm and imparting tension on his pancreas. Chapter 9 described how somatomized content put the valve between the last part of my small intestine and the beginning of the colon into spasm and landed me in the ER with abdominal pain.

Chapter 8 explained how the brain automatically dumps emotions in the tissue whenever we get an overload. Overloads are subjective and situational. In other words, what we take in stride most days may be too much to handle when we are feeling poorly, having a bad day, or are busy or in danger. It may be hard to recognize our own overreacting at times, but we've all had the experience of seeing someone else over-reacting to something we've said. Perhaps, the over-reaction had as much to do with what was going on with the person at the time as our ineptitude or inappropriateness.

Chapter 10 explains how symptoms and illness can sometimes be buried treasure because they get our attention and induce us to roll up our sleeves and get to work, when we might not otherwise. When this is the case and we find and address the associated emotional trauma, we not only start to get well, but we may be on our way toward deeper, more lasting health.

As I mentioned in the Introduction, most of the hundreds of chronic pain patients I saw in the United States Air Force hospital pain clinic had three things in common: 1) they were extremely self-critical; 2) they believed that in some important way they were inadequate, not good enough, or flawed; and 3) they had an unusual band of fascial tension around their respiratory diaphragm. Once they turned the first two around and we freed up that diaphragmatic fascial band, their pain diminished rapidly and often disappeared altogether.

This is why, before starting treatments, I set my intention to find content quickly if doing so is in the patient's best interest. So often, releasing content is the quickest, easiest, and most economical path to health. When patients understand somatomization but aren't willing to work with their content, I'm forced to consider resistance, our next topic.

CHAPTER 12

Resistance

Arguably, resistance deserves its own book. It's that common, problematic, and multi-faceted. While it assumes many forms, resistance falls into two main categories: 1) fear of getting healthy/ attachment to illness, and 2) fear of re-experiencing painful feelings. These categories are not mutually exclusive. Indeed, both may be in play. We all have some resistance—otherwise, all of us would be healing spontaneously around the clock. Therefore, resistance is usually more a question of degree.

Some resistance is obvious: for example, where a patient has a financial or emotional stake in staying ill. Most of us have heard of people who didn't begin to heal until their injury lawsuit or worker's comp claim settled. In the military, some patients won't get better until their medical discharge and percent of disability/ associated compensation has been finalized.

Resistance to Health and Attachment to Illness

Patients may pine for good health and believe that getting well is their number one priority, without realizing or admitting the extent to which some part of them may be attached to their illness or injury. Carolyn Myss, the medical intuitive, believes that this is true with many of those suffering from chronic health challenges. In some way, being ill works for them: it may have gotten them attention, helped them avoid unpleasant chores, or allowed them to duck responsibility. Fearful about losing that, they have become attached to their illness.

Illness arises for many reasons: confusion, environmental exposure, genetics, learning/programming, emotional and spiritual upsets, injuries, accidents, infections, and bad habits. Whatever the cause, as unpleasant as illness is, if we've been ill for months or years, it's a known entity, something we're grown accustomed to and have become good at, which is why being sick can feel safe. Akin to boarding an accelerating train, the idea of having to jump back into life, by contrast, can be scary.

Furthermore, if we were healthy once, look where that got us: sick. Why would we want to risk having our hopes, plans, and dreams dashed all over again? For example, Dr. Upledger told the story of a Parisian beauty who had been paralyzed in a car accident and stuck in a coma for several months. Fearing she would never be able to dance with handsome young men again, some part of her refused to regain consciousness. Knowing that our cerebral cortex and amygdala are always awake, even during a coma, Dr. Upledger explained that, even if some of the activities she had previously enjoyed might no longer be possible, there were still other things to live for. Apparently, he was convincing: she regained consciousness and began the long road to recovery.

It Serves a Purpose

As the above story suggests, when there is resistance, whatever the cause, that's where we have to start. We have to understand why it's there. Once we know what function it serves. we may be able to help the patient devise a healthier way of dealing with the underlying issues. In this sense, the process is like breaking a spell.

Resistance does not imply that we are flawed or inadequate, and it isn't necessarily willful, conscious, or bad. Typically, it served a constructive purpose at some time. Most resistance stems from our need for safety. Survival, both physical and emotional, is our number one priority. How could it be otherwise? Until we feel safe, we must resist. Therefore, manual therapists treat resistance as a potential ally to win over, not an enemy to defeat. This begins with the recognition that the resistance also seeks what's best for the patient.

The Three Ps

Sometimes what keeps a patient stuck is less resistance and more an attitude or belief. It's not that we wouldn't like our challenge to go away, we just don't think it's possible. Thanks to the power of the human mind, what we think tends to be what we experience. Paul St. John, the creator of Neuromuscular Therapy, identified three beliefs that keep us ill, namely that our illness is 1) personal, 2) pervasive, or 3) permanent. Personal means that we believe our case of X is the mother of all cases of X, or our illness Y is illness Y on steroids. Pervasive means that we believe our illness affects every aspect of our life (work, play, cooking, socializing, sex, etc.) Permanent means that we believe that there is no cure, for example, that our illness is age-related, genetic, or fatal.

When meeting a patient with one of these beliefs, his strategy was to create doubt. To show how that works, he told a story about a new patient, a man in his 70s. When St. John introduced himself and asked how he could help, the patient immediately said, "I've a bum knee, my right knee, and there's nothing you can do for it."

"Why are you here then?" St. John asked.

Shrugging, the man gave an irritated, dismissive look at his wife. "She thinks you can help me. She dragged me in here."

St. John then asked, "Why do you think I can't help you?"

"My knee is 72 years old," said the patient.

St. John thought about that for a moment and then asked, "And how is the other knee?"

"Fine," said the patient. "No problem."

"And how old is it?" asked St. John.

The patient looked aghast, as if St. John was an idiot. "Same age as the right. Why?"

St. John had gently disproven the patient's theory that his knee problem was age-related and therefore permanent. St. John's next challenge was to learn why the patient was so attached to having a bum knee. That cleared the path for treatment and the possibility of healing. Of course, these beliefs are not always so apparent and accessible. Often, they are buried in the tissues. That makes them no less powerful. Wherever they are, manual therapy can help find them and bring them to the patient's awareness where they can be addressed.

Occasionally, a new patient shows up in my office dragging a hand-truck of medical records. This is not promising. It raises the possibility that all three Ps may be present. The patient may be signaling that he's been everywhere and tried everything and I should give up before we even begin. That stack of records may be a trophy: they have the mother-of-all cases of their particular challenge; the specialists' notes, test results, and x-rays to prove it. The fact that he drags this symbol and proof of his illness everywhere he goes strongly suggests that he is fully attached to and identified and enmeshed with his health challenge.

To varying degrees, we are all prone to attachment. Once, while a colleague was working on me, I made some comment about "my PTSD." About a minute later, she stopped what she was doing and said, "Did you just say 'My PTSD'? Why are you so attached to it? Why do you want to personalize it and make it yours? Would you be willing to let it go?"

I loved her for saying that. "Sure. Why not?"

Compared to dragging around several cartons of medical records on a hand-truck, my slip of the tongue may seem insignificant but, from a practical perspective, it's pathological. Indeed, 65 years was a long time to drag around a security blanket. My colleague had reminded me how easy it is to become attached to illness without realizing it and the importance and power of words.

Many of us grew up on societal and familial sick-making messages. Typically, they suggest that some flaw—stupidity, ugliness, laziness, and so forth—is responsible for our suffering. Variants include messages that we are somehow physically, mentally, emotionally, or intellectually flawed. It's as if some person doled out roles in a play. Many of us heard one or more of these growing up and internalized them. For example, "You have a weak chest." "You always get ear-infections." "Your immune system has always been weak." "You were colicky as a baby." "You've always had a sensitive stomach." "You're way too sensitive." "You're just as crazy as your mom." "Stupid, aren't you?"

There may have been a grain of truth to the message initially. We may have had or displayed one or more of these symptoms or attributes at some point, but the constant reminding was neither helpful nor healthy. The more important question, why, is rarely raised or answered. If there ever was one, the initial symptom, problem, proclivity, or reaction may have nothing to do with us or our constitution. Furthermore, the implication that what once was shall always be is false. People outgrow childhood challenges all the time.

In a Family Way

Epigenetics, the study of gene activation and deactivation, shows that genes are continually getting turned on and off, without any changes to the sequencing of the gene's DNA. (The latter would be mutations). Factors that result in gene expression or silencing include diet, exercise, relationships, geography, occupation, stress, lifestyle, beliefs and feelings. Therefore, many health challenges that run in families may not in fact result from bad genes as is often assumed but may be learned behaviors that we've been coached in from an early age. The learning originates with some form of "Illness X runs in our family" message repeated over and over, *ad nauseam*.

The underlying message is: "This is how our family reacts to life—and you will, too. It's your responsibility to carry on this wonderful tradition, if you know what's good for you/if you want to be a member of this family in good standing." Given our hard-wired, mammalian need to belong to the group no matter how toxic the group or some of its members may be, it's a wonder that more of us aren't sick.

One reason that these messages are so unhealthy is that they imply that a particular illness is inescapable, a *fait accompli*; it's not a matter of if, but when. If we hear messages like this, day in and day out, year after year, guess what? That's probably what we're going to experience. Talk about a self-fulfilling prophecy!

For example, a patient complained of persistent TemporoMandibular Joint (TMJ) pain. She said that TemporoMandibular Joint Dysfunction (TMD) ran in her family on the female side. She said that during holiday meals, only the men talked at the table. The women remained silent except for their jaws, which clicked audibly throughout the meal as they chewed. Even the jaws of those women who married into the family did this. They all suffered from TMD, too.

Though TMD is significantly more common in women than men, I'm guessing that TMD is not a sex-linked trait, but a cultural one. Many cultures and families encourage men to have and express opinions while discouraging women from doing so. This alone could generate anger, frustration, a sense of inequality and unfairness, all of which could result in tension in the jaw, and eventually clicking and TMD. It's possible that the women in my patient's family were conversing or protesting in the only way permitted: clacking their jaws.

One of the reasons that humans hold stress or tension in their jaws is biological: teeth are weapons, designed for biting. Indeed, one of the very first things an infant must learn is not to bite the hand, or breast, that feeds it. Next, it must learn not to bite the dog, siblings, or playmates. Youngsters who fail to learn these rules get booted out of preschool, kindergarten, and birthday parties. Adults generally have those instincts under control, but any conflict between what we would like to express (especially frustration or anger) but feel we can't or shouldn't, is likely to manifest as jaw tension, pain, and dysfunction. Humans aren't the only species that snarl, gnash their teeth, or pop their jaws when under stress. Indeed, dogs and bears are famous for it.

Unless we believe our illness is our inheritance, that we owe it to our family to carry on this great tradition, or that there is something noble or even saintly about taking on everyone else's stuff, we can probably change and choose health.

Two More Ps: Profitable and Punishment

Sometimes people stay ill in the hopes of gaining a financial reward or to punish themselves or someone else. Arguably, there may be no greater attachment to illness than a belief that profit lies in it. In the introduction to this chapter, we mentioned situations like pending lawsuits and divorces, criminal trials, insurance settlements, worker comp claims, and disability settlements. Common to all is the belief that if the ailment persists, the patient stands to profit, financially or otherwise.

In cases like these, all the king's horses and all the king's men can't put a patient back together again, at least not until the case is resolved and the financial terms are finalized.

Working for the US Air Force, I encountered service men and women who had decided that their symptoms and diagnoses were their key to an early, honorable discharge. (Lest readers assume that this is the norm, it isn't. A far larger number who seem unfit for service due to pain and injury insisted on continuing in the ranks as long as possible at a high personal cost. Using pain and illness to avoid their obligations is surprisingly rare, given what these men and women have to do.) In any event, no matter what we tried, with personnel who wanted out, symptoms rarely budged. When future compensation is based on the severity of symptoms and the degree of disability, the reluctance to improve or show improvement is understandable. In such cases, there is an argument for postponing treatment until everything settles.

Personal flaw messages can damage our relationship with ourselves. Many kids who had horrific childhoods were told that their mistreatment was their fault, that they brought it on themselves by being "bad," "evil," "just like so-and-so," and so forth. To survive physically, emotionally, and even mentally, children often accept these rationales. Unfortunately, doing so can turn us into self-punishers and produce ironclad resistance. In the process of avoiding the pain of the earlier experiences, we may create new painful experiences. Ironclad is not synonymous with indestructible. Resistance can melt.

Making different choices may offer a way out of chronic suffering. About 15 years ago, I attended a talk by Palden Gyatso (*Autobiography of a Tibetan Monk*). Imprisoned for 33 years by the Chinese for proclaiming Tibet's independence, he was tortured almost daily by the prison guards, many of whom were Tibetan like him. He was angry at his torturers at first. Once, he even spat on one, hoping the guard would kill him in retaliation. When that failed to work, he remembered his Buddhist training and began to practice Tonglen which consists of taking in the torturers' anger and returning it as compassion.

Tonglen didn't stop the torture, but it did lessen Palden's experience of pain. Ironically, several of his torturers noticed the change and asked him to become their spiritual guide. After listening to Palden, I realized that holding on to my childhood traumas was only punishing me while simultaneously impairing my ability to help my patients. That realization helped me move forward.

Many of us survived childhood by thinking, rather than feeling. Whether the challenge arose from Dad's drinking, Mom's narcissism, a sibling's rage, someone's mental illness, the family or neighborhood bully, this kind of history tends to make us over-reliant on thinking throughout our lives. Brilliant as our thinking may be, however, if we could think our way to health, we probably wouldn't be reading this chapter. When we tire of the high personal cost of over-thinking and begin moving towards health, we can find ourselves on a rich spiritual path.

Too often, we are encouraged to hammer our symptoms into submission using willpower or failing that, with supplements, medicine, surgery, or self-medication with drugs, alcohol, sex, or consumer therapy. As often as not, however, symptoms are our body's or our spirit's way of getting our attention and leading us to awaken to our own true nature. Similarly, resistance may be a clue that something important is at play. Perhaps we are approaching the issues that will lead us to health, which can be scary if all we've known is illness and pain.

In Chapter 10, I wrote about a patient who felt so bad about a crime he'd committed that he was determined to punish himself for the rest of his days. While I understand his remorse, guilt, even shame, his choosing self-punishment suggests a deep spiritual injury.

Self-punishment may have an outward target. We may believe that by staying sick we can make someone else pay or otherwise suffer, perhaps a partner, friend, or family member dependent upon us or saddled with our care—crazy as that may sound to those who value health above all things. The ultimate combination of punishment and self-punishment is suicide.

Resistance to Re-experiencing Emotional Pain

Sigmund Freud saw resistance as the patient's natural and often unconscious inclination to avoid the pain associated with old memories. We may or may not remember the original emotional trauma consciously, though our unconscious does. Ironically, with this type of resistance, our attachment to avoiding pain produces it in another form: our physical illness and suffering.

In *Working with the Dreambody*, Arnold Mindell, PhD, wrote, "Some people would rather die than revisit early childhood traumas." Mindell understood resistance and had great sympathy for those experiencing it. He explained that being left to cry one's self to sleep for the first time without being held and comforted might seem like no big deal to an adult. However, for an infant completely dependent on others for survival and comfort, this situation amounted to the termination of life support and would be viewed as life-threatening. It could produce such overwhelming abandonment, vulnerability, and helplessness that many of us would rather die than revisit the associated terror.

On many levels, living in mortal fear of something that we nonetheless survived may seem crazy, but that does nothing to diminish its power. Indeed, this is a classic example of how somatomized content mires us in a dysfunctional past. Moreover, since our ego wants to retain control at all cost, it tries to convince us that we can't handle these old traumas. Too often, it succeeds.

Obviously, we have all experienced overpowering emotions. But that was then, and we survived. With the passage of time, most of us grow wiser, stronger, and have a better support group than we did as children. All of this leaves us much better equipped to revisit old traumas and slay the associated emotional dragons.

Nonetheless, many adults avoid revisiting childhood trauma, believing that we've already processed the trauma or that revisiting the past is pointless or emotionally dangerous. These attitudes are wonderfully conveyed in expressions such as "This-discussion-is-over!" and "Been there, done that." Were this actually true, meeting the trauma one more time shouldn't be a big problem.

For readers who think that fear of re-traumatization may be at the root of their resistance, this book is filled with stories that show how easy it is to let go of old emotional trauma, even some very nasty stuff, without any re-traumatization. Chapters 9 and 10 contain several worth reading.

Frequently, I encounter patients who insist they have worked through all their issues. It's possible, if unlikely. However, since somatomization is an unconscious, automatic process, they can't truly release the content until they stumble upon it in the tissues.

In manual therapy, content can pop up at any time. When it does, it's because the patient is ready to handle it. It also means that some health-seeking part of the patient has overcome the inertia associated with resistance. If the patient is ready, asking, "What's right about this (illness or symptom) that I'm not getting?" will summon the content into conscious awareness.

There is another potential source of resistance and illness. To survive or win parental acceptance and approval, traumatized children can take on their parent's attitudes and see the world through their eyes. The resultant "trances" completely color perception making it impossible for the person to experience reality objectively. These trances can make it impossible for the person to see how they are creating their own life and health challenges. Treatment may require psychotherapy. Readers can learn more about this in Stephen Wolinsky's *The Dark Side of the Inner Child.*

It's worth remembering that the nervous system does not distinguish physical pain from emotional. In other words, what seems like a horrific physical problem may just be some content clamoring for attention. Unfortunately, not understanding this, patients and their doctors often attack the messenger, the nervous system. The associated drugs and procedures not only damage arguably the most important system in the body, thus impairing its ability to keep us safe and healthy, but they also rob us of opportunities for emotional and spiritual growth.

We have now looked at some of the common types of restrictions behind many health challenges. Having explored the potential benefits of approaching chronic health challenges as manifestations of mechanical restrictions, somatomized content, and possibly resistance, you may well wonder if manual therapy might be able to prevent illness and injuries. The answer is yes! as you'll learn in the next chapter.

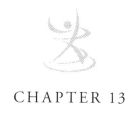

CHAPTER 13

Giant Steps: Prevention and Optimization

In a sense, prevention and health optimization are opposite sides of the same coin. Prevention involves eliminating factors contributing to illness, while optimization removes obstacles to wellness. Inside the body, those factors and obstacles include mechanical restrictions, somatomized content, and toxins. Eventually, this removal process produces an absence of illness; in other words, wellness. If continued after symptoms disappear, manual therapy increasingly segues from prevention into optimization.

Prevention

Since all restrictions eventually cause disease, by finding and releasing them, manual therapy meets the definition of prevention in the strictest sense. This is especially true when we free up restrictions years or decades before symptoms arise. Releasing restrictions and buried content also leaves us more vital.

As previously noted, the American Medical Association reports that stress causes 80% of the illness in the United States.

By finding and evicting content, freeing up our tissues, and showing us that healing is possible, manual therapy reduces our stress and bolsters our resistance to it, thereby preventing a great deal of illness. Furthermore, by teaching us how to listen to, honor, and work with our bodies, manual therapy also provides us with a host of self-care tools that are also preventive.

Here's a partial list of conditions that manual therapy may prevent:

Chronic pain and nerve problems

Breathing challenges like asthma, bronchitis, and pneumonia

Infections, allergies, and auto-immune problems

Digestive challenges: (GERD), hiatal hernia, gastritis, and Irritable Bowel Syndrome

Gall stones, appendicitis, and adrenal challenges

Musculoskeletal, joint and spinal challenges

Circulatory challenges and hypertension

Cognitive, sleep, and behavioral, challenges like ADD/ADHD, failure to thrive

Endocrine and reproductive challenges

Some cancers and tumors

Chapter 3 described how manual therapy boosts the immune system, thereby helping it prevent and fight infection and repair damage. When we use the immune system to remove debris and toxins from tissues and restore normal tissue tone and fluid circulation, we may be preventing malignancy and other diseases. When we use it to remove scar tissue and plaque from arteries, we make the heart's job easier, and we may prevent hypertension and heart attacks. By freeing up restrictions on internal organs, blood vessels, and nerves, we may prevent joint injuries and degeneration and joint replacement surgeries. The list goes on.

Chapter 9 described how one-way valves in the gastrointestinal tract also act as emotional circuit breakers. When we find one of them in spasm and release it, depending on which valve it is, we may be preventing any number of digestive challenges, including appendicitis, gallbladder attack, diabetes, and GERD. That chapter included two stories related to these valves. In one, we managed to lower dangerously high blood sugar levels. In the other, a physician's palpations inadvertently reset my ileocecal valve, possibly preventing appendicitis.

My favorite prevention story occurred about 20 years ago when I began to experience some vague, intermittent sensations in my brain. These were just under the skull, beneath the joint that separates the right side of the top of my head from the left (the sagittal suture between the left and right parietal bones). The sensations were nothing dramatic, just a little tension for ten or twenty minutes a couple times a day for several weeks, but they were troubling.

The most troubling thing was their coming from inside my head. Nobody wants a brain tumor. Like most people experiencing troubling symptoms, I wondered about them when I felt them and tried to put them out of my mind the rest of the time. In short, I hoped they'd disappear and tried to ignore them. I thought manual therapy might help, but wasn't sure who could help me locally. After nearly two months of this, an opportunity to go to Vancouver, BC, arose on very short notice. Remembering an advertisement in our practitioner directory, I called Soma Therapy Center, hoping they could squeeze me in.

The therapeutic relationship is said to begin with the initial phone call. My voice set off something of a crisis on the other end of the line. Somehow, the therapist who answered intuited that I was critically in need of care. Unfortunately, I was arriving in three days and would only be there over the weekend. The phone answerer had me wait while she conferred with her colleagues. Upon returning, she said that the consensus was that my situation was urgent and offered to juggle patients so that all four therapists could work on me at once in a double session. Thinking of those strange sensations in my head, I readily agreed.

While manual therapy is typically done by one therapist on one patient at a time, advanced practitioners train in and sometimes provide multiple-therapist treatments. It's impossible to quantify exactly, but each additional therapist can raise the therapeutic power several fold, perhaps exponentially, especially when all the therapists speak the same therapeutic language (in this case the cranial rhythm) and work together well.

Owing to stress, resistance, anticipation, flying, or some combination, I came down with a killer cold the night before my treatment. My sinuses throbbed. My throat burned. After a miserable, nearly sleepless night, I called the clinic first thing to explain the situation and give my practitioners the opportunity to avoid exposing themselves to my contagion. They would not hear of it. Therefore, I went.

Individually, while the others were out of the treatment room, each practitioner did their hands-on assessment. Once all had finished, they asked me if it would be okay for them to compare notes in front of me. The similarity in their findings was remarkable: a restriction deep in my head, a bunch of restrictions on the left side of my neck, one on my right femur, and one on the left side of my rib cage, which was nearly rigid. Zannah Steiner, the lead therapist, told me that her sense was that my falx cerebri was starting to calcify. She added that she had never treated this before but had seen it recently in a cadaver dissection class.

The falx cerebri divides the brain into left and right hemispheres. One of three intracranial membranes, the falx provides several critical services, it: 1) holds the cranial bones together; 2) accommodates movement; and 3) contains the brain's drainage system for spent CSF and blood, metabolic wastes, and toxins. The flexibility allows for the continuous expansion and contraction of the head necessitated by the filling and emptying of cerebrospinal fluid. The falx communicates tensions and dysfunction between the cranial bones, brain, spinal cord, and body. Finally, it serves as a motion-dampening container, protecting our tofu-like brains from damage when we move or stop suddenly. A rigid falx cannot provide these essential services, and mine was turning to bone.

Zannah said, "The situation with your falx is akin to a slow-moving medical emergency. You've said that you get CranioSacral Therapy fairly often so those gentler techniques haven't resolved this problem. My osteopathic training includes some direct releases. For the falx, they can be very painful, but I think it will be worth it. For a few minutes, it's really going to hurt. Are you willing to give it a try?"

Without knowing exactly what was in store, I was. Indeed, I was feeling extremely lucky to have stumbled upon these therapists. Off we went: me on the table with four, highly-trained, highly-experienced, super-compassionate practitioners latched on wherever their assessments told them to be. Donning an exam glove, Zannah told me, "The key to freeing up the falx is the ethmoid (a small bone behind the nose). However, since there is no direct access to the ethmoid, I'm going to use the maxilla (the bone the upper teeth are attached to) to reach it."

I nodded an okay, and off she went. She'd been honest. Her thumb bearing down on my upper jaw produced several minutes of excruciating pain. Since her pressure was directed at the bone mere millimeters from the tear ducts, I couldn't have helped crying if my life had depended on it.

Even when there are only two practitioners, multiple hands-on therapy makes it nearly impossible for the patient to track everything going on simultaneously. I could feel the hands, of course, and initially had a sense of what each therapist was working, but soon gave up trying to figure out what they were collectively doing. As the therapists reported in about my tissues, I marveled at their ability to feel what was going on in my body. After a few minutes, my falx softened, the other therapists reported changes in the tissues under their hands, my cranial rhythm came back on, and we all took a short breather.

As soon as we'd dusted ourselves off, we went back to work. This time, I quickly went into a therapeutic position. Described in Chapter 6, these are positions that the body was in when it was injured. Reverting to those positions provides avenues of exit for the stored force. My head was cranked to the left, left ear almost touching my left shoulder, neck nearly bent in half.

And there I stayed. Though I had no recollection of having ever been in this position before and no images or memories arose, the position was so extreme that I knew that the therapists couldn't have put me in it without breaking my neck and paralyzing or killing me. For 45 minutes, the only changes were minute corrections that intensified the position and left me even more boxed in, as impossible as that seemed.

Pain-wise, this seemed like a cakewalk compared to the earlier falx-freeing. Thinking that I could withstand this position for hours, if necessary, the ridiculousness of that prospect dawned on me: My airway was obstructed, almost pinched off. I could hardly breathe. Hands were pressing heavily on my chest. My head felt squashed. My neck should have been broken. Finally, allowing myself to experience the physical discomfort, I laughed. This was some cosmic joke, and I was paying four practitioners for it.

The laughter quickly segued into tears. There was but one possible, inescapable explanation: Someone had tried very hard to break my neck. I allowed myself to feel the associated physical pain. While I processed this, my neck began to spontaneously unwind from its extreme position. After a couple of minutes, the unwinding slowed and then stopped, leaving my neck and head in a nearly neutral, anatomical position. The four therapists compared notes about my cranial rhythm and the condition of the tissues at their various stations. All normal. They balanced me out, and the session was over.

In the ensuing weeks and months, there were no hiccups, no flashbacks, or crises. Either I didn't need to re-experience the original trauma, or wasn't ready to. However, that session did help me make sense of many things: childhood depression, my first marriage, and the car accident and whiplash that propelled me into manual therapy, etc. More importantly, I came away with more self-compassion. In any event, those troubling symptoms just under the skull at the top of my brain have never returned. Knock on wood.

While these two anecdotes may seem like they're mostly about tissue memory and buried trauma, they're really about prevention. Just as the medical resident's palpation may have prevented me from having appendicitis and spared me from having an appendectomy, I'm certain that reversing that calcification in my falx prevented some serious neurological and cognitive impairments.

This is precisely the problem when talking about prevention: Since it didn't happen, we can't prove we've prevented anything. Sure, we know how certain illnesses and syndromes usually progress, but when we intervene, we can never be absolutely certain what would've happened had we not. This truism applies not just to manual therapy, but also to medicine, chiropractic, acupuncture, even to life in general.

What I do know is that those four women reversed the calcification of my falx cerebri and released a nasty restriction from my neck. Those weird sensations near the sagittal suture in the middle of my head have not returned. I'm confident that they prevented some degenerative, currently incurable brain challenge like Parkinsons, Alzheimer's, dementia, or senility. Take your pick.

If those four women hadn't found and addressed that calcification, I probably wouldn't be here today, 20 years later, hiking up mountains, cross country skiing, picking berries, writing, helping patients. Living. Instead, I would have experienced an increasing number of bizarre symptoms, starting with headaches, as the brain is not built for bashing up against a bony barrier. If the onset continued at a leisurely pace, these symptoms would probably have left a lot of physicians scratching their heads and telling me not to worry. Eventually, an MRI would probably have revealed the ossification, and some doctor would have told me that they couldn't tell me why but I had an inoperable, degenerative, and ultimately terminal brain condition. They couldn't tell me how long I would have to live or what kind of symptoms I would experience, but I should get my affairs in order.

Instead, those four women fixed the problem the same day they found it, without any tests, drugs, or surgery. A few minutes of physical pain allowed me to dodge a major bullet at a fraction of an MRI's cost. That would have been followed by the months and tens of thousands of dollars of additional tests and specialist visits, most likely leading to a hopeless prognosis—unless, of course, I was lucky enough to encounter a doctor who was aware of CranioSacral Therapy (CST) or cranial osteopathy and willing to suggest I give it a try.

If a manual therapist eliminates a lung restriction or restores adequate blood supply to the cranium, can he or she claim to have prevented migraines, degeneration of the cervical and lumbar spines, damage to the medulla oblongata, or thyroid problems? Probably not, though he or she may well have. For any given challenge, there are innumerable potential causes. For example, restoring adequate blood supply to the brain can prevent headaches, migraines, and cognitive issues; endocrine problems; chronic muscular tension in the neck and shoulders and spinal degeneration; and circulatory challenges in the abdomen and extremities. I've seen this sort of treatment resolve those kinds of symptoms, even though we can't prove that by treating a restricted carotid artery we've prevented disc degeneration and bone spurs, but we probably have. Therefore, we can content ourselves knowing that chronically tight shoulders, necks, and skulls immediately relax when we do and the patient looks younger and more vital and reports feeling considerably better.

The same goes for lung restrictions. We can feel them jamming the head down on the neck and compressing the cervical vertebrae and brain stem on each inhalation. We can feel this stop after we've released the lung restrictions. For me, that's proof enough that we've prevented some serious pathology.

When we help a patient end years of being stuck in fight-or-flight, we may resolve chronic digestive, cognitive, immune, musculoskeletal, sleep, and adrenal challenges. If those symptoms haven't yet reached the patient's awareness, absent our intervention, they almost certainly would eventually. Therefore, we can say we've cut short a pathological process before any damage has been detected and improved the function and vitality of the central nervous system and probably every other system, organ, and tissue in the body. That's early detection and prevention.

Every day, manual therapy reverses the course of serious disease processes, with no undesirable side effects or collateral damage. And with its access to immune cells that eliminate damaged tissues and replace them with healthy tissues, manual therapy can facilitate and accelerate subsequent healing. Manual therapy empowers patients to take charge of their health rather than be helpless bystanders or even victims.

It is impossible to overstate the role that the mind plays in health and illness. And it's worth remembering that the mind is not restricted to our head, but encompasses our entire body. The issues, beliefs, and attitudes that we've unconsciously parked in our tissues continuously broadcast pathological messages to our brain and the rest of our body. Therefore, finding and releasing those pathological messages has huge ramifications for preventing illness and promoting health.

These are a few of the reasons why I believe that manual therapy has virtually unlimited prevention potential and why it can dramatically reduce the need for drugs and more invasive and expensive procedures. But don't take my word for it: see for yourself. You'll feel better and, even if you never know exactly what you've prevented, you can be confident that being healthier will help you dodge significant disease.

Optimization

As wonderful and desirable as wellness may be, something even better is possible: optimal health. Admittedly, optimal health sounds a little nebulous. How do we know what it is? How do we know when we've attained it? The moment we experience an improvement in our health, we have positioned ourselves for the next improvement, and the next. We have raised the bar for what is possible. In this sense, optimal health is a little like the ever-retreating pot of gold at the end of the rainbow. But the big difference is that we can feel the improvement, acknowledge it, revel in it, appreciate it, and improve upon it.

Athletics is a good example of optimization. With effort, focus, and dedication, an athlete can improve his performance. In the world of competitive sports, records are broken frequently. We see this in track & field and swimming, where performance can be precisely measured. We also see it in sports like hockey, football, basketball, figure skating, and snowboarding, gymnastics, and climbing, which have their own metrics. In every age group and from amateur to pro, people keep breaking records, redefining what is possible, for themselves, their sport, and for our species.

It's important to differentiate between the process—optimization—and the goal, optimal health. Arguably, this entire book is about that process. However, I wrote it for two reasons: first, to inform readers about how their bodies work and second, to encourage readers to embrace the possibility of attaining optimal health, especially those who'd resigned themselves to being ill for the remainder of their lives because they'd never heard of manual therapy and did not understand their body's mechanical needs.

Optimal health is subjective, differing for each individual, based on their genetics, history, circumstances, and psyche. Lifestyle, exercise, relationships, and nutrition also play roles in optimization. Meditation, yoga, acupuncture, and other practices can all help, but none can compete with manual therapy for eliminating the physical restrictions that, in so many different ways, keep us anchored in dysfunctional pasts and pathological presents.

Many of us have been fortunate enough to have felt on top of the world at some point in our lives, if only briefly. It may have been when we were kids or teens. Remembering exactly what that felt like may be a challenge, especially if those moments were fleeting and those days are long gone. But it needn't be all downhill from this moment forward.

Though she's experienced enough physical and emotional trauma to fill several lifetimes, Venus tells me that each morning she wakes up in love with life. Is that a form of health optimization? You bet. It gives her a resiliency to life's challenges, whatever their nature. And being in love with life attracts good things, in the form of prosperity, abundance, and people capable of sharing love.

When we release a restriction in the chest and the patient suddenly exclaims, "Wow, I can breathe again!" she is getting a foretaste of what optimal health might feel like. The same thing is true when we free up a restriction on the heart and a patient feels lighter and her entire chest softening, relaxing, opening. Or when we free up a kidney and years of low back pain suddenly stops.

When a patient discovers that he's always felt inadequate, unworthy, or unloved or that he is stuck in self-judgment, or is his own worst critic, a different possibility opens for him, should he choose. While this realization may be painful, it probably is not nearly so painful as has been his daily experience. That pain cannot compete with the exciting possibility of a whole new way of being.

Mind you, even if the symptoms don't return, feeling on top of the world may be short-lived because that sense of relief and freedom soon becomes the new normal. Although the novelty may wear off, however, the improvement need not. The experience nevertheless awakens us and is a stepping stone on the path toward optimal health.

Here is my optimization story: I've been an athlete for more than 50 years. For decades, my favorite summer exercise had been hiking up the mountains overlooking Anchorage, Alaska as quickly as I could comfortably. As far as aging is concerned, we are told that slowing down is inevitable, and we are programmed to expect it. During my 66th summer, however, my times improved by 25%. My standard hike, a 1500-foot vertical climb that had previously taken 40 minutes, required only 30 minutes with the same effort. The 1900-foot climb that used to take 60 minutes took only 45. Etc. Indeed, my only complaint was that there weren't 25% higher replacement peaks readily available from the trailhead because I love being in the mountains and I love the exercise, and all things being equal, longer is better. Who would have thought it? What else is possible? Can I go faster next year, with the same effort? Seems unlikely, but… why not?

I hadn't lost any weight or changed it to muscle. I hadn't increased the intensity of my efforts. The hills hadn't shrunk: they are just as tall and steep as they were 20 years ago. I can only attribute that improvement to manual therapy, mindfulness, and the accompanying emotional and spiritual work. Thanks to that breathing exercise in the Appendix, I'm breathing better. Thanks to mindfulness, those old negatives play less frequently and I am more present. Who can predict what benefits and efficiencies will flow from that!

In 1969, Carole King and Gerry Goffin wrote a song advising us to take a giant step outside our mind. "Remember that feeling as a child, when you woke up, and morning smiled? It's time to feel like that again." Taj Mahal immortalized those lyrics in his album Giant Step. Whatever your goal, manual therapy can help you take that step.

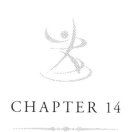

CHAPTER 14

A Typical Treatment

Readers unfamiliar with manual therapy might be curious about what a session is like and what the patient experiences. This chapter should answer some of those questions. Of course, there is no such thing as a typical treatment because no two patients, no two therapists, and no two treatments on the same person even from the same therapist are exactly alike. Each patient is forever changing in terms of needs, especially if she's receiving bodywork. Similarly, no two practitioners are exactly alike, even if their training is similar. Therefore, the therapeutic dance between each practitioner and patient continuously evolves.

How We Begin: A Typical First Session

As mentioned before, the therapeutic relationship begins when a new patient calls to see if we are a good fit and if so, schedule their first appointment. New patients fill out a questionnaire about their health history, complaints, goals and contact information prior to treatment as they would at a doctor's. I won't look at what they've written before treating, but I must determine if there are any contraindications to treatment or parts of the body we need to avoid because of recent injury, surgery, infection, or artificial devices like pacemakers, stents, or mesh.

Some patients expect only a consultation on their first visit. While we could easily pass an hour talking, exploring the patient's history, situation, and symptoms, as important as their story may be, manual therapy is about what the tissues have to say. Furthermore, we'll usually make more progress if we keep the patient focused in her body. In many ways, we don't need to know why she's come and what she hopes to gain. While we care a great deal about their history, story, and goals, our primary job is to find out what the body's most pressing needs are and address them. We do that by listening to the body with our hands and going where we're drawn.

Whole Body Assessment

I ground myself and set my intent to find what's most important for this patient on this day. With the patient standing in his stocking feet, I'll gently lay my palm on top of his head and silently call the weakness or restriction up into my hands. This is called general listening. Placing my other hand over the spot where I'm drawn helps me pinpoint the most pressing restriction.

Restrictions can be anywhere and in any type of tissue, such as bone, joint, tendon, ligament, cartilage, muscle, blood vessels, nerves, or internal organs. If it's in the head, for example, it could be a bone, an intracranial membrane, blood vessel, or in the brain itself. The restriction's location and nature help determine the treatment technique, but all are surprisingly gentle, even when a restriction is deep in the body and protected by bony structures.

For example, when general and local listening drew me to a patient's chest, we found two restrictions behind the sternum, one near the top of his heart on the right, and one behind his heart, also on the right, but a little lower. When I asked, he said he'd been injured in a car accident. When the airbag failed to inflate, he'd slammed into the shoulder harness.

Most of the time, I treat patients on the massage table. They are face-up and fully clothed. Usually, face-up is more comfortable than face down for them and I can hear and track their facial expressions better. If I need to access their abdomen or back, I explain what I would like to do and ask permission to work under their shirt or trouser waistband.

Comfort, on all levels, is critical. Physical comfort is important because many patients are in pain. Addressing that may involve placing pillows under the head and knees. Unless the room is exceptionally warm, I'll usually provide a blanket because metabolism often slows during a session, and if patients don't feel toasty, they won't fully relax. Indeed, any kind of stress or discomfort significantly limits how much we can accomplish.

I'll continue to assess the tissues with my hands. Ankles, heels, shins, thighs, hips, ribs, shoulders, and head. I'll check to make sure feet, knees, and hips are level and symmetrical—often they aren't. Is the trunk straight? Often there are offsets. Are the shoulders even? Is the neck centered on the shoulders? Is the head straight or crooked? Are the eyes level or offset? Ditto with the ears and jaw. These are visual clues to underlying restrictions, or the lack thereof.

All the while, I'm listening with my hands for fascial tensions and the expansion and contraction of the patient's lungs. Are right and left lungs inflating equally, simultaneously, and smoothly? Often, the answer is no. Often, inflation begins in one lung first, or one lung may not inflate as much as the other. Often, the thorax barely expands, and most of the breathing is in the abdomen. How do the abdominal viscera and the heart respond? The answers are all clues.

Cupping the back of his head in my palms, I'll listen to the widening and narrowing of his head associated with the production and reabsorption of Cerebrospinal Fluid (CSF). Is it fast or slow, strong or weak, equal on both sides, full and expansive or faint and empty? At about this point, I'll ask the patient what brought him in? What's going on? If I hear a litany of complaints and problems, I'll ask him to name his top priority.

Meanwhile, I'm already segueing from assessing into treating. The distinction is somewhat arbitrary if only in that the simple act of observing a system changes it. This is especially true with the human body, which is so receptive to what others think. Furthermore, I can't be in another person's space without changing his energy and body. The very act of listening with my hands wakes up the patient's tissues. Even as I treat, I'm continuously monitoring the patient's body and tissues, and not just where I'm working. I'm looking for connections, clues, signs of response and change everywhere.

This street runs both ways: while I'm focused on my patient, my patient's body is checking me out, too, and for good reason. I am in my patient's personal space to a degree that few other people are ever allowed. When patients are lying down and I'm standing, I tower over them. Even perched on my stool, I'm still head and shoulders above them. Developed over eons, the patient's survival instinct recognizes the implicit imbalance and the resultant vulnerability and keeps asking silently, "Are you sure this is such a good idea?"

Even for people whose interactions with other humans have been mostly positive, submitting to this power imbalance and physical intimacy requires incredible trust and continuous verification. Many of my patients have experienced horrific treatment from the very people that they most loved, trusted, and depended upon. This leaves them all the more guarded.

No matter how many positive things a new patient may have heard about me, we've only known each other for a few minutes. Therefore, of course, the patient's nervous system is continuously monitoring the quality of my touch and presence to decide how safe she is, how safe I am, and what she can safely show me.

I often begin treating at the top of the neck. If so, I'll try to free up the joint between the occipital bone at the back of the head and the first cervical vertebrae. This is the occipital-atlas joint, or O-A for short. Ironically, this is one of the most vulnerable places in the entire body. For starters, it's where our spider-sense is, where we feel a tingle, look across the room or street, and see that someone whose presence we weren't aware of is watching us. Back in the day, it was also the place where predators would have grabbed us in their jaws. So many vital and vulnerable structures are located here, all it would take is one crunch, one blow, and we're dead. In other words, I'm on thin ice here.

It's also the place where many people tend to store tension. For example, when we spend time staring at computer screens or print, talking, or doing precise tasks with our hands like typing and texting, the resultant tension lands in the back of our head. Put one hand back there, close your eyes and move them left to right. Can you feel the tissue beneath your hand move? Now talk. Can you feel the tissue move? How many hours of looking, talking, and keyboarding do you figure you do in an average day?

My intention in starting here isn't to stir up those primal defense mechanisms and put my patient into full alert. Instead, I'm assessing the amount of tension and how quickly it will release. I'm also gathering information about the relationship between the patient's head and his body. Are the two relatively independent and therefore functioning well, or are they locked together? Is the dominant tension in the head or in the body?

Just by looking, I already know if my patient has any neck at all. Many do not. Like the turtle, many have pulled their heads into their shells. I'll learn if there is an imbalance in tension in the neck from side to side, and if there is, I'll gain a sense of whether it's coming from the head, the neck, or down in the body. This simple release provides an opportunity to assess the entire bodymind and provide some therapy.

Meanwhile, I may make an occasional comment or ask a relevant question. I'm looking for short answers because the patient's talking will add to the tension at the base of their occiput and slow down or arrest a release. Despite the neck's vulnerability, patients love the O-A release, precisely because of the tension carried there. Releasing the O-A may improve the venous return from the brain by 50 percent, which means that we may improve the Central Nervous System's (CNS) arterial supply and function.

If a patient entrusts me with this most vulnerable part of his anatomy, we're probably going to be able to get a lot of work done right from the get-go. Otherwise, we're going to have to take it slow until we've established a sense of safety. For some, feeling safe may be a huge improvement over their normal experience. Indeed, opening to the possibility that they could feel safe may be the biggest and most important step they've ever taken toward healing.

If the O-A joint of an adult opens easily, the patient has probably had manual therapy before and has probably never experienced whiplash or other severe neck trauma. There is another compelling reason to start out at the O-A: I will know immediately if he has significant lung restrictions because I will feel the head jamming down on his neck on each inhalation if he does.

A Quart Low

If the O-A joint doesn't free up after a few minutes, there will be a good reason. Although the tensions may provide some clues as to where the problem originates, I probably won't know yet. I'll leave the O-A for now. But the resistance to opening is a critical piece of information. It could be a restriction in or affecting the spinal cord or it could be that the brain's blood supply is inadequate. The latter is exceedingly common and except in the most extreme cases, rarely diagnosed. Often it means that one or more of the four arteries supplying blood to the brain is challenged. Either the arteries have been injured, have plaque deposits, are being compressed by some other tissue, or are being compromised by content.

If I find an arterial shortfall to the brain, I'm going to investigate and treat it. This might consume an entire first session. In addition to the arteries of the neck, on the heart, aorta, and subclavian arteries may be involved in the work. Indeed, the restriction or restrictions causing the problem could be anywhere: in the head, neck, thorax, abdomen, leg, or arm. We'll go wherever the tissues take us. Even though I may start on the head, that doesn't mean that I'll stay there. It's possible to feel a restriction in one of the arms or one of the legs from the head. If we do, that's probably where we need to go.

Patients often ask how I can find a restriction on a well-armored structure like the heart or brain. The reason I can find restrictions through the ribs or skull is simple. Restrictions pull on surrounding tissues. We can feel those pulls and follow them. We have fascia's elastic component to thank for that. It attracts our hands to the restriction. When the pull stops, we know we've arrived or are very close. At that point, we ease up on the pressure and allow the tissues to make subtle adjustments as we locate the restriction even more precisely in three dimensions. Often, that is enough to occasion a release. If not, we have lots of other ways to obtain a release, all of them gentle.

Once I find the restriction and direct my patient's attention to it, he often feels it, too. Or he may instead feel the paradoxical relaxation that occurs as we approach and arrive at the restriction, even before it releases. When the restriction finally releases, both of us often simultaneously feel an opening or expansion at the site and in the surrounding tissues or region.

During any treatment, I always hope to address part or all of the patient's chief complaint. However, this is often not possible in a single treatment. The problem may be complicated or longstanding. Frequently it is not the body's highest priority. Even if we make little or no progress on the patient's priority, patients usually feel appreciably better. We've probably released half a dozen or more restrictions. Nearly every release will leave the patient feeling more relaxed, more open, lighter, softer.

If it was a colon restriction, for example, the patient's abdomen may feel looser. Her hip might move better. If we free up one or both kidneys, her lower back may flatten against the table and her pain may ease. If it was a lung or heart restriction, she might be breathing more fully with less effort, and her chest will feel more open and relaxed. The joint between her first cervical vertebrae and her head may be much freer.

If she wasn't getting enough arterial blood to the brain and we address that, her head will feel softer. The CNS will work better, and that will help every other system in the body. By the same token, once the CNS's needs for blood are addressed, other organs and tissues that may have been clamoring for more blood for years might finally get their requisitions filled. Patients may experience this as warmth in the extremities. If her cranial rhythm had been weak, it will be much stronger, and the head will sit much straighter on the shoulders.

Unless we've missed something or the patient is intent on re-injury, releases usually last. For months or even years. This is because we don't force releases. Techniques are gentle; we go with the tissues. Manual therapists don't try to impart or impose some ideal configuration to the spine or any other structure. Realigning the spine with adjustment after adjustment or massaging tight muscles again and again may bring temporary relief, but, as often as not, it may be undercutting the body's best efforts to deal with those restrictions. I learned this from having had whiplash and in the course of my training.

If a restriction doesn't release after a few minutes and the patient is willing, I will talk directly to the patient's body. The patients tell me the answers they hear in their minds. I could guess, but why would I want to do that? Every tissue in our body is highly intelligent. The more we can tap into that intelligence, the faster we can find out what the problem is and what needs to happen to correct it. I talk to tissues and symptoms because it works. The more I can engage a patient in her treatment, the better. As much as I love spending time with my patients, I don't want them to spend the rest of their lives on my table.

No two manual therapists work exactly alike. But most of us share abiding respect for the human body, considerable training in anatomy and physiology, considerable curiosity and compassion, and an ability to feel what's going on in the tissues and find and release restrictions.

Most of my patients are relatively healthy. For example, they aren't suffering from congestive heart failure, kidney disease, or diabetes. If they've had cancer, it's probably in remission. But their complaints are serious: chronic pain, headaches and migraines; allergies and other immune challenges; and respiratory, digestive, circulatory, cognitive and developmental challenges. Many are stuck in fight-or-flight, some have anxiety or PTSD. While most are able to work, everything they tackle is more of a challenge than it would otherwise be. Many are unable to participate in activities that they enjoyed formerly.

Many of my patients have been all through the medical system and alternative therapies with little or no relief. Some have been told, "It's all in your head." Others, "There's nothing else we can do for you." Or, "You're going to have this problem for the rest of your life so get used to it." And worse. After months of making little or no progress, some just stopped going to wherever it was. In many cases, their case wasn't hopeless. Their doctors simply didn't understand the body's mechanical needs or lacked the time and techniques to address them.

Over the decades, I've become convinced that most of us have within us everything we need to heal and get well. We just haven't found the person who can help us find it, or found the restriction that has created our challenge. Occasionally, I get to treat people hospitalized with acute conditions, such as the results of a car accident or fall. Even though the hospital bed and the monitors and drips and catheters make it a challenge to physically access the patient, sometimes the improvement in a patient's appearance is so dramatic that I thank my lucky stars on my way home. I know that there are tens of thousands of manual therapists around the world who feel the way I do about their work and their patients.

A Stitch in Time

If you're thinking that this manual therapy sounds great, but you don't have any real challenges that you know of, so you'll check it out later, think again. Since we live on a gravity-rich planet, we all have restrictions. Some of us have hundreds of them. All restrictions are pathogenic. In other words, they will eventually compromise your health.

For example, earlier, we talked about arterial insufficiency for the brain, how common it is, and how most of us who have it are unaware. If that includes you, that single problem alone will wreak havoc on your CNS and impact every other system in the body. Symptoms could include headaches and migraines or cognitive, endocrine, immune challenges, and thermal challenges, chronic fatigue, anxiety, and on and on. Basically, any problem in the body could be a symptom of arterial insufficiency to the brain. If that is the root of the problem, a manual therapist can probably correct it in a few minutes.

Why wait for full-blown symptoms to arise before we seek treatment, when a little manual maintenance could prevent the problem and its collateral damage? For example, by freeing up restrictions on nerves and blood vessels and eliminating adhesions and scar tissue on internal organs, manual therapy can help us move more functionally and reduce wear and tear on the articular surfaces of our joints. This allows us to enjoy our favorite activities while avoiding hip, knee, shoulder, and back surgery. The same can be said for releasing restrictions in the lungs and respiratory diaphragm. That may be one of the most important ways to maintain healthy spines and lifestyles and avoid discectomies and spinal fusions. Finally, as discussed earlier, manual therapy can prevent, delay, or lessen the severity of the loss of mental acuity attributed to aging.

The next chapter is for those readers ready to find a manual therapist.

How to Find and What to Look For in a Manual Therapist

Finding a manual therapist who is right for you may take a little work, just as finding a primary care physician would. If you live in affluent parts of the country, for example, a major metropolitan area, the urban Northeast, Northern California, Pacific Northwest, and Florida and are mobile (able to drive or take mass transit), you'll have many options. Less so in rural parts of the Midwest and South. This person may end up knowing much more about you than your doctor or almost anyone else, so once you've narrowed the field, find someone that you're comfortable with.

Selecting a manual therapist is essentially a two-step process, with some overlap. After finding out who is out there from on-line directories, the winnowing down begins. During this phase, the primary focus is on their qualifications: training, experience, and proficiency. Therapist profiles and websites can be helpful, but at some point, you're going to have to talk to the therapist and ask some questions. Thus, begins the second phase of the process through which you gain a sense of the person: Are they safe, experienced treating your specific challenges, open to working with you? If not, can they suggest someone else better suited to help you? To be a therapeutic experience, this has to work for both of you, so don't be afraid to ask questions and have the therapist clarify any answers that you don't understand.

Assuming you end up having a treatment or three, you should very soon be able to tell whether this is the right manual therapist for you. If not, don't be afraid to move on. Always, always trust your intuition.

The following discussion assumes the reader has access to the internet and the practitioner directory. Www.iahp.com lists nearly everyone in the world who has ever had one or more workshops in CranioSacral Therapy, Visceral Manipulation, and several allied modalities.

Training Type

Please, please, keep in mind that everything that follows in this chapter is a generalization. Since this book focuses on CranioSacral Therapy and Visceral Manipulation, what follows is largely a discussion about how to find practitioners with these trainings and, if you are fortunate enough to live in proximity to several or more, how to choose among them.

Most practitioners specialize in either Cranial or Visceral work, though many advanced practitioners have some training in both. Cranial and Visceral are quite different and tend to attract different types of practitioners. In general, CranioSacral practitioners tend to be guided by the Cranial Rhythm and the Inner Physician and, compared to Visceral Manipulation practitioners, are more likely to do emotional release work. Guided by fascial tensions, Visceral Manipulation practitioners tend to be more anatomically precise and are likely to do a considerable amount of tissue listening and testing before treating. Since they often retest after each release to determine the extent to which the body has changed, Visceral patients may be getting on and off the table several times during a treatment.

Training Amount

Ideally, you'll look for a provider who has had at least three courses in either modality. This level of training suggests at least a passing interest in and rudimentary understanding of the modality. This is in addition to whatever training was required for their licensure: usually 600-1100 hours for massage therapists, three years for physical therapists, four for chiropractors, seven or more years for medical doctors. If your challenge is complicated or your history is complex, look for a practitioner with at least six (6) workshops. In the CranioSacral world, this usually includes significant training in emotional release work. In the Visceral world, this would mean that she's had training in treating most of the internal organs and an understanding of how all of them fit and work together.

Given the variety of backgrounds, interests, and skills practitioners offer, it's extremely difficult to say which modality is better for what. However, if you have an immune problem, you might do better with a practitioner who has had CranioSacral Therapy and the Immune Response (CSIR), or if something is going on in your head, The Brain Speaks class (TBS). If you have a nerve or vascular problem, you might do better with a Visceral practitioner, especially if they've had training in Neural Manipulation (which is an offshoot of Dr. Barral's Visceral work). (At the outset, I warned about generalizations because these distinctions break down with advanced practitioners.)

Nearly every field (Massage Therapy, Physical Therapy, Chiropractic, and so on) requires that practitioners receive a minimum number of hours of continuing education every year to keep their licenses current. Therefore, if someone in the directory has only one or two classes listed after his name, you'll have to probe to find out if he is new to the field and excited about manual therapy or has just taken a class because he was curious or needed the credits. You'll have to ask if he's incorporating these new techniques into his treatments. Going from how we were trained and what we've always done to something new is a big step for some of us and some of our patients. Not everyone manages to take that step. It's not uncommon, however, for someone with just a class or two to be proficient. Therefore, if the therapist sounds confident and you believe him (and that's your only convenient option), this person is worth a try.

Training Providers

Although there are other forms of CranioSacral Therapy, I recommend seeking practitioners trained through the Upledger Institute (UI)/International Association of Healthcare Educators. Similarly, For Visceral practitioners, I would seek those trained by the Barral Institute (BI). Both UI and BI maintain the highest standards for their instructors and continually upgrade their curricula, course content, and materials. Nearly thirty years ago, when I took my first Cranial class, I was struck by the instructor's professionalism and clarity. Assisting with classes frequently, I'm continually impressed by the constant refinement of the courses and instruction.

Alternatives

Should there be no UI/BI trained practitioners in your area, your best bet might be an Osteopathic Physician who specializes in manual therapy (most do very little or no manual therapy, preferring to practice medicine). Some osteopathic manipulations are high force, and most American osteopaths probably won't be doing overt emotional release work. You'll have to decide what you need. In the US, very few osteopaths will have taken a UI CST class because Upledger makes them start at the beginning with the first level (CS1), even if they've been doing manual therapy and craniosacral releases for years. (The primary rationale for this requirement is to teach light touch.) Abroad, it's common to find osteopaths taking and teaching Visceral and Cranial classes.

An increasing number of Rolfers (Structural Integration) are training in Visceral Manipulation but won't be listed in the IAHP directory because their VM training is not directly through the BI—although their instructors have been trained and approved by Dr. Barral. Many Rolfers have specialized in treating the musculoskeletal system and typically don't do emotional release work, but there are exceptions.

The UI directory also lists practitioners trained in several other allied manual therapies which might be well suited for your issue. Another option might be practitioners trained in Myofascial Release (MFR), an early offshoot of CranioSacral Therapy started by Dr. Upledger's research colleague John Barnes, PT. Some MFR-trained practitioners specialize in emotional release, others in gentle fascial stretching.

If the IAHP directory does not list any practitioners convenient to your location and none of the other options mentioned pan out, word-of-mouth may be your only choice locally. Certainly, it's worth considering any practitioner with whom friends, family members, or acquaintances have had good experiences.

Ideally, it's nice to be able to work with a manual therapist locally. Failing that, if you visit some major city several times a year, you may be able to find a practitioner there. Finally, there are several CranioSacral and Visceral Manipulation therapy centers in the US and Canada worth considering—and more sprouting up in Europe, South America, Asia and Australia and New Zealand. The Upledger Institute Clinic in Palm Beach Gardens, Florida, offers everything from single treatments to intensive week-long multi-practitioner programs for people with major challenges like spinal cord and brain injuries to strokes. Run by one of the most senior Upledger CranioSacral Instructors, Integrative Intentions has similar offerings in Truth or Consequences, New Mexico.

Proficiency

UI and BI-trained practitioners mostly come from the ranks of physical, massage, speech, and occupational therapists, chiropractors, and acupuncturists. Each background brings distinct differences in training, expertise, philosophy, and benefits. Both UI and BI offer two levels of credentialing: the technique, which might be considered journeyman, and the diplomate, which is expert. Both involve written and hands on examinations and assure competency and understanding. Any current instructor in either modality will be highly competent and have diplomate status.

The bottom line is that practitioners should be sufficiently skilled to be able to feel what's going on in your tissues and communicate it to you. (What they say may or may not resonate with your experience, but it should not feel wrong.)

Experience

Experience involves how long the therapist has been in practice, how busy her practice has been, and what type it is. Obviously, someone who has been practicing full-time in a busy practice for a number of years is going to have much more experience than someone who has been doing manual therapy on the side for the same number of years. Similarly, full-time means different things to different practitioners. You can ask how many patients they treat in an average week and how many weeks they treat each year.

There are also different types of practices and patient populations. For example, some physical therapists specialize in helping people recover from fractures, joint injuries, and surgeries while others focus on helping people with strokes or brain injuries. Some therapists work mostly with adults, others with children. If the prospective patient is an infant, toddler, or child, you'll need a practitioner trained and specializing in pediatric manual therapy. Ask prospective manual therapists to describe their practice: do they specialize in any types of patients or challenges? What are their primary professional interests? How do they like to work? What's a typical treatment like?

For a simple problem, someone who has only had one or two classes might be all you need. Certainly, when I was just starting out and had had only a couple of classes, I was able to help people with some pretty serious problems. If you have the option, however, go up the food chain.

As you narrow your search and begin talking to, meeting, and actually working with practitioners, pay increasing attention to intangibles such as personality, maturity, life experience, things that in addition to training, experience, and manual skills are likely to contribute to your having a therapeutic experience. These factors will help you decide whether to schedule an appointment or, having had a treatment, continue.

Safety

Safety is the bottom line for any therapeutic relationship. Your practitioner must be able to create and maintain appropriate physical, social, and professional boundaries by being clear about roles, the therapeutic relationship, confidentiality, and time and money matters. These are not negotiable.

This is only the foundation. In a therapeutic relationship, the therapist holds the greater share of the power and must be able to minimize this imbalance, while maximizing the patient's collaboration. Practitioners must be capable of honoring, erecting, recognizing, and maintaining your boundaries for you. They must be able and willing to say no, gracefully.

Safety is critical as it enables patients to focus on their issues. Part of feeling safe stems from the therapist's ability to withhold judgment. We've all made mistakes and done stupid things. Look for practitioners who accept you the way you are, regardless, no matter how desperate you may be to improve.

Compassionate

Look for practitioners who care about you and others. You will know this by what they say about you and others; how they treat coworkers, employees, and animals; how serious they are about their work; and what they choose to do in their spare time.

Most jurisdictions require practitioners to be licensed and approved by a state or national professional board. Therefore, most practitioners have some sort of credential, usually indicated by letters after their name. Indeed, the sheer number can be a bit baffling. For example, more than half a dozen describe massage therapists. These include Licensed Massage Therapists (LMT), Certified Massage Therapist (CMT), and Registered

Massage Therapist (RMT). An acupuncturist might be Licensed (L.Ac) or a Doctor of Oriental Medicine (DOM). PT stands for Physical Therapist, often suggesting Master's level training, PTA is a Physical Therapy Assistant. Nowadays, freshly minted PTs are usually DPTs, meaning they have a doctorate or PhD in Physical Therapy, usually involving three years training, original research, and a dissertation. If the practitioner is listed in the IAHP.com directory, any acronyms and what they stand for should be searchable there. All of the IAHP courses they have completed will be listed there, too. Click on any acronym and a description should pop up.

While not a guarantee, credentials imply a certain amount of training, winnowing, and professional recognition. A therapist should be able to explain each credential listed after his name, what training was involved, where and when it was obtained, and what it signifies. Patients should always feel free to question a therapist about his training and background and should expect honest, detailed answers. Anything less may be a red flag.

To a certain extent, manual therapy training and practice self-selects for many of these characteristics. We tend to know who is right for us when we meet them. This is a felt sense, stemming from feeling welcome, accepted, supported, and empowered. We feel their confidence and skill. Taken together, these things can provide as sense of trust. When embarking on a journey through a strange and confusing land, we need and deserve the best companions and guides.

CHAPTER 16

Conclusion

In 1988, I immediately sensed manual therapy's almost unlimited power and potential. If anything, in the three plus decades since, manual therapy has exceeded my expectations many times over. Meanwhile, Dr. Upledger, Dr. Barral, and their colleagues have relentlessly explored and extended the boundaries of the profession. As a result, the unimaginable has become routine. For example, if you'd told me back then that we could eliminate a life-threatening allergy or clear fluid-filled lungs in a few minutes, I wouldn't have believed it. But having seen it and felt the tissues changing, I know it's true.

Most of these anecdotes come from Alaska, where I practiced for thirty years before moving to Oregon. I've concealed the identities of the patients whose stories pepper these pages because, despite its vastness, Alaska resembles a small town in many ways. As a result, Alaskans tend to know their neighbors more than folks in Manhattan or Los Angeles do. Many of my patients know each other.

Ironically, my military patients, who had served to protect my freedoms, were stuck with me, as I was the only massage therapist employed anywhere by the Air Force at that time. The quantity and variety of traumas in many of their bodies forced me to grow as a person and practitioner. Their stories are not in this book, but working with them confirmed what I'd long come to believe: namely, that there are few conditions that manual therapy cannot help. I am so grateful for having had the opportunity to get to know and help those men and women and for their willingness to roll up their sleeves, talk to their bodies, let go of the content we found in their tissues, and decide that they too deserved to be healthy.

Working with them reminded me that most people don't understand their bodies and, as a result, undergo too many tests and procedures and take too many medications that are expensive, intrusive, unnecessary, and ultimately counterproductive. By contrast, so much of what we accomplished came relatively easily. When they expressed surprise at the newfound ease and comfort in their bodies, I would tell them that when we don't like the doodles in our body, removing them is often simply a matter of choice.

Since fear, and especially the fear of the unknown, is so powerful, many of us desire a diagnosis and cling to it once we have it. I suppose there's some comfort in having an explanation for our illness or pain, even if it's not the whole story. But there's no reason to settle for a diagnosis when health might be just around the corner.

GERD is a classic example. Explored in detail in Chapter 3, GERD is often a mechanical issue. Namely, a valve fails to stay closed when it's supposed to. Yet, medicine usually treats GERD as if it were a biochemical challenge needing permanent pharmaceutical management, even though manual therapy may eliminate most cases.

For many challenges, manual therapy offers a get-out-of-jail-free card. And even when it doesn't completely free us from the slammer of pain or illness, it still leaves us healthier and closer to a solution than before. This can't be said about pharmaceuticals, which typically suppress symptoms in lieu of addressing underlying causes, often at the cost of undesirable side effects.

Like medicine, manual therapy is a collaborative process between practitioner and patient, but even more so, because the patient and his or her body are in charge, as opposed to the doctor. Typically, treatments last an hour and most of that time the therapist's hands are on the patient's body. We proceed at the patient's pace. If recovery is an option, the more the patient is involved and invested in the process, the faster recovery will arrive. The opposite is also true: for example, patients involved in lawsuits and worker compensation claims often make little progress until their cases settle—no matter how much treatment they get. This speaks volumes about the power of the mind in matters of health.

Not knowing any better, some patients call me a healer. The simple truth is that we can only heal ourselves. Admittedly, I have many tools and decades of experience to facilitate my patient's healing, but if I leave them believing that their health depends on me, I have done them a huge disservice. Manual therapists create a healing space for our patients and then hang out in it with them. This is sweet indeed; few occupations offer such benefits to its workers. There's a fine line between demystifying manual therapy on the one hand and demonstrating its power and potential on the other. My intention has been to accomplish both.

It still amazes me that one can feel something as subtle as the cranial rhythm. With some of the restrictions I've felt, I'm astounded that those patients can still function. That they can underscores our body's resiliency and built-in ability to compensate. In any event, the fact that the cranial rhythm is palpable throughout the body allows us to find and release restrictions and improve tissue function and fluid exchange.

Similarly, new patients are often amazed to learn that their internal organs have their own innate motions and that we can feel these motions with our hands. This is especially true with the heart and lungs, protected as they are by the ribs, sternum, and spine. And yet, when my hands follow their heart's motility, many patients begin to perceive the movement. When we corner thoracic restrictions, even before we release them, patients can perceive their chests relax and breathing improve. When we release lung or heart restrictions, it's as if we'd turned the clock back decades while simultaneously making it possible for patients to be more present.

Having now learned about fascia, we can understand how a restriction will eventually affect every other cell in that body. On some level, most of us have always known about this connectivity or at least suspected as much. But gaining a felt-sense somehow makes our inter-connectedness that much more real. Knowing that imaging technologies typically used by doctors do not reveal damaged fascia, we can understand why so many patients have been told that their problem must be in their head so get used to it.

Great though it may be, intellectual understanding pales in comparison to feeling a restriction, or its release. The sense of newfound freedom, empowerment, and control can move us from thinking and feeling like a victim to feeling that we have options, good options, where before, at least subconsciously, we may have felt trapped. The notion that much of the entrapment stems from compensation—the body just trying to make the best of the cards it's been dealt—is in itself a revelation, especially for those who've believed that their bodies were stupid.

The fact that the body manifests our thoughts and commands provides an avenue out of chronic illness and challenges, even those that have plagued members of our family for generations. This is our Declaration of Independence from the tyranny of illness.

In the first decades of personal computers (PCs), a new PC would start off great but within months would begin to slow down. This decline resulted from limited storage capacity and the PC's seemingly random parking of fragments of information (data, documents, and applications) across the hard drive. The solution, defragging the hard-drive, essentially reorganized files and applications and went a long way to restoring the computer's original processing speed.

Ironically, our Central Nervous System does something similar with the physical, emotional, and spiritual trauma we encounter in life. These overloads end up in our tissues, increasing entropy. Over the decades this has the effect of transforming us from vital, active homo sapiens children to achy, crotchety slowmo sapiens senior citizens. Since we can't throw ourselves away and buy a new body the way we can with a computer, manual therapy is the best way I know of defragging our body and forestalling many of the ravages of time.

The Access Consciousness® statement "What else is possible?" expresses both gratitude and our ongoing willingness to receive. Furthermore, it acknowledges that we have a choice. For those who assumed they had no choice, this realization marks a critical shift and can provide a solid foundation for health.

For example, when we improve the blood supply to the brain, the physical sensations can be remarkable, whether it's our neck lengthening, shoulders dropping, brain bobbing on a sea of CSF, our head softening, our vision changing, energy rushing down our arms or legs, or tingling all over. But as pleasant as those sensations may be, the real relief stems from the sense that much or all that we thought was carved in stone is built of sand.

As reluctant as we may be initially to look under the hood for emotional content, most patients come to understand that parking content in the tissue is normal and releasing it is easy and safe. Indeed, once they realize that content often holds restrictions and pathology in place and once they experience how easy and painless it is to let go of content, they usually embrace the process. Many begin to hope, as do I, that their complaints are rooted in buried content because releasing them can be the expressway to health. Regardless of whose content it is, how long they've had it, and whether or not they've worked on the associated history consciously, they come to realize that they aren't doing anyone any favors by holding on to it and are only hurting themselves. Talk about liberation through understanding.

The idea that it's possible to find and release mechanical restrictions in the tissues is exciting. However, of all of these revelations, perhaps the most astounding is that patients can talk directly to their tissues and even symptoms. While this conversation can resolve chronic and mysterious health challenges, it also suggests that health is often both a collaborative and elective process between mind and body, with the mind ultimately holding the reins. The underlying message here is that if you don't like the result, change your thinking.

The operant question is, "What's right about this that I'm not getting?" But please, don't ask it while operating equipment or driving. This looking-under-the-hood approach flies directly in the face of victim-thinking and the belief that our health depends largely upon someone or something else: the other driver, our parents, siblings, friends, childhood, spouse, roommate, life-partner, genes, doctors, technology, or drugs.

Of the many examples of the healing power within our grasp, few are as profound or important as our ability to work directly with our immune system to combat infections; eliminate scar tissues, adhesions, plaque, toxins, and toxic emotions; and replace damaged tissue with healthy new tissues. Nothing short of revolutionary and miraculous, our immune system can be the ticket out of autoimmune challenges and chronic illness. Combined with the astonishing advances in medicine, manual therapy can deliver the promised lands of wellness and health optimization.

I hope that the foregoing information and anecdotes have convinced you that there is something to this manual therapy. In thinking about the amazing experiences patients have had over the years, it's tempting to wonder what will be next? The answer is that the next is already here: manual therapists are making new discoveries and introducing powerful new techniques and treatment modalities all the time.

Thanks in part to manual therapy, when it comes to health and healing, it certainly appears that the sky is the limit. My prayer is that you find this to be so. Choose health. Make healthy choices. A santé! To your health!

Interrupted Breathing Exercise to Override the Stress Reflex and Improve Lung Function

Background

As explained earlier, the stress reflex develops at about age 6 months. Like any other reflex, the stress reflex is automatic and beyond conscious control. However, it is possible to use the structures involved to turn the reflex off once it gets triggered. In Chapter 14, I credited this exercise with significantly improving my ability to ascend mountainsides several years ago when I was 66.

Here's What to Do

Take several normal breaths and determine whether it's easier to inhale or exhale. Always work on the easier side. Therefore, if it's easier to exhale, you're going to inhale normally, but briefly and gently interrupt each exhalation from four to six times on each breath cycle. And you're going to do this for a minute or two. Then you can go back and check to see if the challenged side has improved and to see if it's still more challenging than what was initially the easy side.

You can do this as long and as many times a day as you like. Remember, this is not an Olympic breathing competition. The entire exercise should be as gentle and easy as you can make it, including the interruptions.

This technique comes from Ruthie Alon, creator of *Bones for Life* and a student of Moshe Feldenkrais, creator of Feldenkrais. Both are subtle, profound movement therapies.

How This Works

The CNS monitors all bodily activities, including this exercise, which it interprets as an "all 's well." The CNS then turns on the parasympathetic nervous system, using the vagus nerve to relax the respiratory diaphragm, as well as the heart, lungs, and abdominal organs.

APPENDIX B

Standing Kinesiology/Muscle Testing

We are bombarded continuously by information and choices. Weighing it all can be overwhelming, especially if we lack confidence in our intuition. Muscle testing is one approach to sorting through all the input. The most common methods of muscle-testing include sticking one's arm out and having another person push down on it; making a circle with thumb and trigger finger of one hand and then trying to separate thumb and trigger finger or break the circle with a finger of the opposite hand; and then the standing method that we're about to describe. Two other methods spring to mind: one using a pendulum (a rock or crystal suspended from a string) the other, just becoming as present as you can and then seeing if the item or idea makes you feel lighter or brighter (a positive or yes response) or darker or heavier (a negative or no response).

All may be subject to bias. The first, using another person as a tester or helper can inject their bias as well as yours. My personal favorite uses the whole body. It's not foolproof because we all have biases, but I would argue it's as good as any and better than most. While I wouldn't rely on it for a major life decision, for example whether I should marry someone, quit my job, or buy a house, it can be useful for answering simpler yes-no questions, such as: Do I need this supplement? Should I buy this brand? Should I go to the party? For these kinds of decisions, it works pretty well.

Establishing a Frame of Reference/Baseline

Stand in anatomical position, feet parallel and hip distance apart; arms at side; palms facing forward. Relax. Let yourself get grounded. Normally, eyes open. Closed if there are too many visual distractions. Make sure there is no other person or electronic device immediately in your energy field. Give yourself at least four feet, preferably twice that.

Next, ask your body to show you a big YES! And note what happens. Do you start to fall forward, backward, or sideways? If the latter, to which side? Then ask your body to show you a big NO! How does it respond? Ideally, the movement will be diametrically opposed to what it does when it shows you Yes! If so, you now have a frame of reference for answering simple yes-no questions. If not, move and try again. If the response continues to be ambiguous, this probably isn't a good time or place to do standing kinesiology. You may want to try this at home alone the first couple of times with nothing much at stake (for example, no money involved) just to get comfortable with it.

Because our polarity changes from time to time and because our environment can affect our polarity, we must always establish the yes-no baseline before we do any standing kinesiology. This includes reestablishing the base-line if we move more than a few feet from few feet from where we began or if we're around computers and other major electronic devices.

Ask Yes-No Questions

Once you've established a clear-cut baseline, you're ready to ask yes-no questions. You can always test, by asking a question with a known, obvious answer, such as "Are most books printed on paper?"

Be careful about your wording. For example, do not use the word "want," as in "Do I want to go to the dance or do I want more money." Until very recently, "want" mostly meant "lack" as opposed to "desire," and that's how your bodymind will probably hear and interpret it. In such a situation you could use "Do I desire…?" "Would I enjoy…?" "Would I benefit from…?" "Is it in my best interest to…?" Also, remember to ask yes-no questions and not either-or, for example, "Should I stay home tonight?" As opposed to "Should I stay home tonight or go out?"

You may notice that you know the answers to some of your questions as you pose them. That's okay, that's probably your intuition speaking and is probably worth listening to. What you do with the answers, how much credibility you give them, is your choice, as it should be.

Curing Colds and Flu Using Your Immune System Contraindications: If you are emotionally disturbed or suffer from mental illness, do not try this on your own.

Colds, Flu, Infections, and Healing Crises

At the very first sign of a cold, take action. Don't assume it's a cold. Find out. Ask your body if it's a cold or a healing crisis, using a technique like standing kinesiology to get answers from your body. A healing crisis can feel like a cold or injury, but it's just your body's way of releasing old negative energy and toxins. With colds and flu, on the other hand, your immune system is battling pathogens, usually in your respiratory system, sinuses, or intestinal system— all prime areas for dumping emotional overloads.

You can always ask your body if you have a bug/cold, or if the problem is a healing crisis, or both. If it's the latter, ask what you can do to help. You can always take care of thymus and then ask it to clear the emotional and energetic gunk from the affected areas.

Colds are rarely just colds. Pretending otherwise increases the likelihood of a long, miserable slog. At the very least, getting sick suggests that your immune system is less than optimal. Perhaps, your self-care has slipped or your stress levels have elevated or persisted for too long. You may also have stuffed some emotions that are interfering with your immune response. If so, the sooner that you address those issues, the sooner you will recover.

What follows is a step-by-step process. I suggest that you read it over at least once before you start.

The following approach to working with the immune system comes from the late Dr. John Upledger, D.O. His view of your thymus gland and immune system was thoroughly discussed in the Chapter 3 as evidence of the body's intelligence.

Always Take Care of Thymus First

The following may seem a little cumbersome and long, but that's only because I've tried to cover all the possibilities. In practice, and with practice, it's quite simple.

Lie down, if possible, with a pillow under each elbow.

Place the heel of one hand on your upper sternum, and the heel of the other hand atop the first.

Ask thymus if it will talk to you. If you hear a "yes" in your mind, ask it how it is doing. The answer is important. If it has challenges, ask how you can help.

Ask thymus if it has enough space. If the answer is yes, ask if it would like more. Ask thymus to attract your hands wherever they need to go to optimize its space. Even if you don't feel anything, stick with it for five or ten minutes. Even if you can't find and release all the restrictions crowding your thymus, it will appreciate and reward your efforts.

Repeat all of step 1, this time focusing on thymus's blood supply. Ask thymus if its blood supply is adequate. If yes, move on to the next step. If not, ask thymus if the blood shortfall is more physical, emotional, spiritual, or a combination. If the answer is physical or a combination, place your hands over thymus and ask your body to guide or attract your hands wherever they need to go to improve thymus's blood supply. If the problem is emotional, spiritual or a combination, ask your body if it you need to know any more about this at this time. If no, give yourself permission to let go of whatever content is interfering with thymus and its blood supply. If the answer is yes, ask thymus how long the content has been there. Once you get that answer, ask your body to show you a person, place, situation, or event associated with that content. If you get an answer, you can ask if it's your stuff or the other person's, if you need to know anything else about it at this time? If you run into a wall and no answers are forthcoming, don't worry. Just move on. Blood may not be a critical issue, anyway, and thymus will appreciate that you tried

Repeat all of step 1 again, this time focusing on thymus's energy. If thymus wants more energy, invite it to pull all the energy it needs from the universe through your hand. Ask it, "If the energy came in the form of light, what color or colors would be most helpful?" If nothing comes to mind, go with white light, which includes the entire visible spectrum. (If you are really sick or exhausted and there is someone around who is comfortable with this stuff, ask them to help intend the f low of universal energy into your thymus. If that's one bridge too far for them, but they are comfortable with touch ask them to put a few fingers on your sternum and send you some love for a couple of minutes.)

Ask thymus what are the most important things you can do to help it. Usually the answer will be "drink more water, get more exercise, or get more rest/sleep." If you get an answer, be sure to comply. Ignore thymus's advice at your own expense. When thymus is ready to go to work, it will feel bubbly or tingly, as if it were a freshly poured carbonated beverage.

Working with Your Immune System

Now that thymus has been helped, you can work with it. Start by asking thymus to send immune cells to the problem area (lungs, throat, nasal passages, sinuses) to look for any cells or substance that looks out of place or different and report back with a physical description of those cells (shape, color, geometry or other distinguishing characteristics. Any description will be immensely helpful. Think in terms of a kindergartener's refrigerator art.)

Once you get the description, ask thymus to send to the problem area whatever immune cells are most effective for dealing with the cells described.

Give thymus a few minutes to accomplish this.

Re-check: ask thymus if all the cells of that description are gone. If not, or if not sure, (virus and bacteria are very good at morphing and hiding) ask thymus what you can do to help and how long it will take to complete the job.

Check for other pathogens. (Repeat step 1.) If you get a description of another pathogen, repeat steps 2-4.

Ask thymus to repair any damaged tissues, if appropriate (in your best interest).

If your illness is in multiple parts of your body (for example, lungs, upper respiratory tract, sinuses), repeat these steps for each part, as the germs may be different in different parts of the body and your immune system needs an accurate description for each pathogen.

When all done, thank thymus for its help and the immune cells and system for their help. Again, ask thymus what you can do to that would be most helpful. Then, take your medicine! In other words, follow Dr. Thymus's orders!

You can use similar protocols to eliminate adhesions, scar tissue, toxins, and emotional toxins. The beauty of working with thymus is that you don't need to know the names of the various immune cells or what they are good for. Don't rush. A slow methodical approach is best. Give thymus at least a fraction of the hour or three you would have otherwise spent going to the doctors. It may take several sessions to beat your cold. Get in the habit of working with your thymus regularly.

Talking Directly to Your Body: Words of Encouragement and Suggestions

People who are not used to talking directly to their bodies may find it a challenge at first. If this sounds like you, don't despair. If you are willing to let it happen, it probably will, though it may take a while. The ego is accustomed to being in control, and like a child too often indulged, ego may resist taking a backseat.

Assuming you are willing, give your body explicit permission to talk directly to you using your voice. In general, it's best to ask simple yes-no-maybe questions, as they minimize the need for thinking. When it comes to working with our body, thinking is over-rated and can get in the way.

Ask thymus if it will talk to you. If you hear a "yes" or "maybe" in your mind, ask it how it is doing. If it has challenges, ask how you can help. If you hear nothing, go directly to step 3; ask thymus if its energy is adequate. Of all the questions you can ask your body, this is the one that your body is most likely to answer, perhaps because thymus embodies the will and ability to heal.

Appendix D: External Application of Castor Oil Packs for Eliminating Adhesions and Softening Scar Tissues

Scar tissues and adhesions wreak havoc with fascia and the subtle and gross motions of internal organs and the musculoskeletal system. Edgar Cayce, a twentieth century medical intuitive and pioneer, recognized the consequent deleterious effects on our health and advocated the external application of castor oil packs, a simple, if somewhat cumbersome, solution. The following is about external, topical application. Ingesting castor oil is not recommended.

Castor oil (from the castor bean, as opposed for Castrol which is for vehicles) softens scar tissues and dissolves adhesions. Although the deadly poison ricin is also derived from the castor bean, the oil itself is non-toxic. However, since castor oil will carry into your body anything it comes into contact with, the areas to be treated should be free of skin cream, after shave, antiperspirants and the like.

For the same reason, the wool flannel cloth should be washed and dried beforehand. This is because not all sheep fleeces are white as snow and the flannel was probably bleached and dyed during manufacturing.

Castor oil is very gooey and difficult to clean up or wash off once it's been applied or spilled; therefore, it is a good idea to have all the gear required before starting.

Recommended Supplies

A pint or quart of castor oil, preferably organic
A wool flannel (or two sewed together) if the area to be treated is large

Saran wrap to prevent the oil from migrating away from the f flannel, and to help hold it in place

An old towel you no longer care about

Safety pins to hold the pack and towel in place

Plastic bags or sheets to protect bedding and furniture from oil, which will stain

A heating pad or hot water bottle to speed the process of oil penetrating the skin and deep into the body

Witch hazel for topical use, cleanup

Plastic bags to protect surfaces upon which you will set down the oil container Paper towels for cleanup

Access to a hot shower for more thorough cleanup

ZipLoc bag for storing pack in fridge between treatments

Something to read if you won't be napping or meditating

A timer to ensure you don't fall asleep under the heat source and burn yourself.

Give yourself time enough (at least 30 minutes, preferably an hour or more) for preparation. Theoretically, you could leave the pack on all night, if you can protect your bedding and clothing, but be sure to turn off the heating source before falling asleep.

Instructions

Saturate the flannel with oil

Secure it in place

Wrap it with the plastic film

Cover with towel

Lie or sit where you can get comfortable

Apply external heat if you can, being careful not to overdo it and burn yourself, either by using excessive heat, spending too long a time, or any combination.

The oil will soften your skin, even after you've washed it off. The length, number, and frequency of treatments depends on the extent and severity of the scar tissue or adhesions. Several treatments of an hour or more will soften most scars and adhesions sufficiently to allow a manual therapist to free up tissues that had previously been glued together.

SELECTED BIBLIOGRAPHY

Barral, Jean-Pierre and Alain Croibier. *Trauma: An Osteopathic Approach.* Seattle: Eastland Press, 1999.

Barral, Jean-Pierre and Pierre Mercier. *Visceral Manipulation.* Seattle: Eastland Press, 2005.

Barral, Jean-Pierre. *Manual Thermal Evaluation.* Seattle: Eastland Press, 2005.

Barral, Jean-Pierre, Stephen Anderson, and Dan Bensky. *Urogenital Manipulation.* Seattle: Eastland Press, 2006.

Barral, Jean-Pierre and Pierre Mercier. *Visceral Manipulation II.* Seattle: Eastland Press, 2007.

Barral, Jean-Pierre and Alain Croibier. *Manual Therapy for the Peripheral Nerves: Osteopathic Diagnosis and Therapy.* Edinburgh: New York, 2007.

Barral, Jean-Pierre. *Understanding the Messages of Your Body: How to Interpret Physical and Emotional Signals to Achieve Optimal Health.* Berkeley, CA: North Atlantic, 2008.

Barral, Jean-Pierre and Alain Croibier. *Manual Therapy for the Cranial Nerves.* Edinburgh: Elsevier, 2009.

Barral, Jean-Pierre. *Manual Therapy for the Prostate.* Berkeley, CA: North Atlantic Books, 2010.

Barral, Jean-Pierre and Alain Croibier. *Visceral Vascular Manipulations.* Edinburgh: Churchill Livingstone/Elsevier, 2011.

Barral, Jean-Pierre. *The Thorax.* Seattle: Eastland Press, 1994.

Batmanghelidj, F. *Your Body's Many Cries for Water: You're Not Sick; You're Thirsty: Don't Treat Thirst with Medications.* Falls Church, VA: Global Health Solutions, 2008.

Brown, Brené. *Daring Greatly: How the Courage to Be Vulnerable Transforms the Way We Live, Love, Parent, and Lead.* London: Penguin Life, 2015.

Brown, Brené. *The Gifts of Imperfection: Let Go of Who You Think You're Supposed to Be and Embrace Who You Are.* Center City, MN: Hazelden, 2010.

Burmeister, Mary. *Introducing Jin Shin Jyutsu.* Scottsdale, AZ: Jin Shin Jyutsu, Inc., 1981.

Burmeister, Mary and Sue Malinski. *Fun with Happy Hands.* Scottsdale, AZ: Jin Shin Jyutsu, Inc., 1988.

Clifton, D. O., and P. Nelson. *Soar with Your Strengths.* Dell Trade, 1992.

Croibier, Alain, D.O. *From Manual Evaluation to General Diagnosis: Assessing Patient Information before Hands-on Treatment.* Berkeley, CA: North Atlantic Books, 2012.

Feldenkrais, Moshe. *Awareness through Movement: Easy-to-Do Health Exercises to Improve Your Posture, Vision, Imagination, and Personal Awareness.* New York: Harper One, 1990.

Feldenkrais Moshé. *Body & Mature Behavior: A Study of Anxiety, Sex, Gravitation, and Learning.* Berkeley, CA: Somatic Resources, 2005.

Gyatso, Palden and Tsering Shakya. *The Autobiography of a Tibetan Monk.* New York: Grove Press: Ill., Maps; 22 cm., 1997.

Haas, Elson M. *Staying Healthy with the Seasons.* Celestial Arts, 2003.

Harvey, Alison. *A Pathway to Health: How Visceral Manipulation Can Help You.* North Atlantic Books, US, 2010.

Hay, Louise L. *Heal Your Body: The Mental Causes for Physical Illness and the Metaphysical Way to Overcome Them.* Carlsbad, CA: Hay House, 2012.

Hay, Louise L. *You Can Heal Your Life*. Carlsbad, CA: Hay House, 2017.

Johanson, Gregory J., Ron Kurtz, and Charles Chu. *Grace Unfolding: Psychotherapy in the Spirit of the Tao-Te Ching*. Harmony, reprint ed, 1994.

Kaptchuk, Ted J. *The Web That Has No Weaver: Understanding Chinese Medicine*.
New York: McGraw-Hill, 2008.

Kurtz, Ron. *Body-Centered Psychotherapy: the Hakomi Method: The Integrated Use of Mindfulness, Nonviolence, and the Body*. Mendocino, CA: LifeRhythm, 2007.

Levine, Peter A. *Waking the Tiger: Healing Trauma*. Berkeley, CA: North Atlantic Books, 1997.

Lowen, Alexander. *The Language of the Body: Physical Dynamics of Character Structure*. Hinesburg, VT: The Alexander Lowen Foundation, 2012.

Lowen, Alexander, Leslie Lowen, and Walter Skalecki. *The Way to Vibrant Health: A Manual of Bioenergetic Exercises*. Hinesberg, VT: Alexander Lowen Foundation, 2012.

Lowen, Frank. *The Roots and Philosophy of Dynamic Manual Interface: Manual Therapy to Awaken the Inner Healer*. Berkeley, CA: North Atlantic Books, 2011.

Mindell, Arnold. *Dreaming While Awake: Techniques for 24-Hour Lucid Dreaming*. Charlottesville, VA: Hampton Roads, 2002.
Mindell, Arnold. *Working with the Dreaming Body*. Portland, OR: Lao Tse Press, 2014.

Neff, Kristin. *Self-Compassion: Stop Beating Yourself Up and Leave Insecurity Behind*. New York: William Morrow, 2015.

Perry, Bruce Duncan, and Maia Szalavitz. *The Boy Who Was Raised as a Dog: and Other Stories from a Child Psychiatrist's Notebook: What Traumatized Children Can Teach Us about Loss, Love, and Healing*. Basic Books, 2017.

Reese, Mark. *Moshe Feldenkrais: A Life in Movement*. San Rafael, CA: Feldenkrais Press, 2012.

Stevens, Robert Tennyson, Gregg Braden, Shabari Lynda Bird, and José Ricardo Fuentes. *Conscious Language, the Logos of Now: The Discovery, Code and Upgrade to Our New Conscious Human Operating System*. Asheville, NC: Mastery Systems, 2007.

Teeguarden, Iona and Duina Pierluigi. *A Complete Guide to Acupressure: Jin Shin Do*. Idyllwild, CA: Jin Shin Do Foundation, 2003.

Teeguarden, Iona. *The Joy of Feeling: Bodymind Acupressure, Jin Shin Do*. Idyllwild, CA.: Jin Shin Do Foundation, 2007.

Upledger, John E., and Vredevoogd, J.D. *CranioSacral Therapy*. Chicago, IL. Eastland Press, 1983.

Upledger, John E. *Craniosacral Therapy II: beyond the Dura*. Seattle: Eastland Press, 1987.

Upledger, John E. *Craniosacral Therapy SomatoEmotional Release: Your Inner Physician and You*. Palm Beach Gardens, FL: UI Enterprises, 1991.

Upledger, John E. *Craniosacral Therapy: Touchstone for Natural Healing*. Berkeley, CA: North Atlantic Books, 2001.

Upledger, John E. *SomatoEmotional Release: Deciphering the Language of Life*. Berkeley, CA: North Atlantic Books, 2003.

Upledger, John E. and Jon D. Vredevoogd. *Craniosacral Therapy*. Seattle: Eastland Press, 1984.

Van der Kolk, Bessel A. *The Body Keeps the Score: Brain, Mind, and Body in the Healing of Trauma*. New York: Penguin Books, 2015.

Wanveer, Tad. *Brain Stars: Glia illuminating craniosacral therapy*. Palm Beach Gardens, FL: Upledger Productions, 2015.

Wolinsky, Stephen. *The Dark Side of the Inner Child: The Next Step*. Norfolk, CT: Bramble Books, 1993.

GLOSSARY

ACEs	Adverse Childhood Experiences
CNS	Central Nervous System
CSF	CerebroSpinal Fluid
CST	CranioSacral Therapy
GERD	Gastro Esophageal Reflux Disease
GI	Gastrointestinal
PRS	Primary Respiratory System
RAS	Reticular Activating System
SIDS	Sudden Infant Death Syndrome
SER	SomatoEmotional Release
SOT	SacroOccipital Technique
TIA	Transient Ischemic Attack
TMJ	Temporomandibular Joint
TMD	Temporomandibular Joint Dysfunction
TCM	Traditional Chinese Medicine

ACKNOWLEDGEMENTS

The idea for this book came before the new millennium, but I made little progress until Dennis Vitrella lit a fire under my keyboard in 2014. Absent Dennis, I'd still be working on the outline. Thank you, Dennis and John Matthew Upledger for all you did for all of us.

Thanks also to: Angeles Scougall Vitrella and the Vitrella's former graphic design and publishing teammates (Phyllis and Robert O'Hair, Anne Pujalte, and Michael Caswell) for their generous assistance with an early draft. Lan Sluder for his comments on that draft and its prospects and for his invaluable insights on the publishing business Melanie McKay, PhD, for your copy-editing and ringing endorsement. Kevin Bailey, PhD for your friendship, encouragement, and modeling what being a successful author requires.

I have several types of teachers to thank. First, are all those who've encouraged my writing these past fifty years. Those no longer with us include Leland T. Johnson, Michael A. Decamp, Barclay Johnson, and John Unterecker. Those still extant include Dexter Newton, Joseph Dupras, PhD, Charlene Avallone, PhD, and Roger Whitlock, PhD.

Secondly are my patients who have shown me time and again that healing is possible. Journeying together, you have taught me courage, fortitude, hope. May we always experience our essence: perfect, whole, complete.

I've been fortunate in having learned from some of the greatest bodyworkers and manual therapists. These include the late John Upledger, D.O, popularizer of CranioSacral Therapy, Susan D. Pinto, PhD; Tim Hutton, PhD., Suzanne Scurlock, Signy Erickson, D.C., Judith Bradley, Zannah Steiner, D.O. and her former team. Jean-Pierre Barral, D.O., creator of Visceral Manipulation and his primary collaborator, Alain Croibier, D.O.; Gail Wexler, Dee Dettmann Ahern, Peter Coppola, and Annabel Mackenzie. Like those already mentioned, my Alaskan mentor Maury Oswald, DO, embodies everything I value: Simply being in his presence, people start feeling better and then, with all his training, knowledge, and clinical experience, the doctor appears.

My formal education in the field began with Iona Marsaa Teeguarden and her Jin Shin Do® BodyMind Acupressure instructors. Much of what I've learned about the psyche stems from several counselors: Bill Wolf, PhD; David Sandberg, PhD; the late Ron Kurtz, PhD, and that magician, Connie Roseman, MS, RN, LPC. Finally, Gail French's Feldenkrais and Bones For Life® teachings enabled me to skate-ski on ice and survive a 15-foot fall onto a road.

Too numerous to mention, my classmates and colleagues have been a wonderful source of support, inspiration, and healing for three decades, especially Barb Carlin, Linda Gill, Sandra Upton, Cathy Teich, and Alisa Eliot.

Most importantly, I must thank my wife, Lauri J. Adams, for her patience, support, generosity, and companionship these 30 years. You are a miracle.

INDEX

Printed in the United States
by Baker & Taylor Publisher Services